C000128246

Emergency Airway Manage...

Emergency Airway Management

Edited by

Jonathan Benger
United Bristol Healthcare Trust, UK

Jerry Nolan
Royal United Hospital, Bath, UK

and

Mike Clancy
Southampton General Hospital, UK

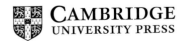

CAMBRIDGE UNIVERSITY PRESS
Cambridge, New York, Melbourne, Madrid, Cape Town, Singapore, São Paulo, Delhi

Cambridge University Press
The Edinburgh Building, Cambridge CB2 8RU, UK

Published in the United States of America by Cambridge University Press, New York

www.cambridge.org
Information on this title: www.cambridge.org/9780521727297

November 2008

Printed in the United Kingdom at the University Press, Cambridge

A catalogue record for this publication is available from the British Library

Library of Congress Cataloging-in-Publication Data

Emergency airway management / edited by Jonathan Benger, Jerry Nolan,
and Mike Clancy.
   p. ; cm.
  Includes bibliographical references and index.
  ISBN 978-0-521-72729-7 (pbk.)
1. Respiratory emergencies.   2. Respiratory intensive care.   3. Airway (Medicine)
I. Benger, Jonathan.   II. Nolan, Jerry.   III. Clancy, Mike.
[DNLM: 1. Airway Obstruction–therapy.   2. Intubation, Intratracheal–methods. 3. Emergencies.
WF 145 E53 2009]
  RC735.R48E48 2009
  616.2′00428–dc22

                                                                2008029601

ISBN 978-0-521-72729-7 paperback

Contents

Contents

Contributors

Jonathan Benger
Consultant in Emergency Medicine, United Bristol Healthcare Trust. Professor of Emergency Care, University of the West of England, UK.

Stephen Bush
Consultant in Emergency Medicine, St. James's University Hospital, Leeds, UK.

Mike Clancy
Consultant in Emergency Medicine, Southampton General Hospital, Southampton, UK.

Andy Eynon
Consultant in Intensive Care, Wessex Neurological Centre, Southampton General Hospital, Southampton, UK.

Colin Graham
Professor in Emergency Medicine, Accident and Emergency Medicine Academic Unit, Chinese University of Hong Kong.

Alasdair Gray
Consultant and Honorary Reader in Emergency Medicine, Royal Infirmary of Edinburgh, UK.

Carl Gwinnutt
Consultant in Anaesthesia, Salford Royal Foundation Trust, Salford, UK.

Simon Leigh-Smith
Consultant in Emergency Medicine, Defence Medical Services, UK.

David Lockey
Consultant in Anaesthesia and Intensive Care, Frenchay Hospital, Bristol, UK.

Nikki Maran
Consultant in Anaesthesia, Royal Infirmary of Edinburgh, UK.

Dermot McKeown
Consultant in Anaesthesia and Intensive Care, Royal Infirmary of Edinburgh, UK.

Patrick Nee
Consultant in Emergency Medicine and Intensive Care, Whiston Hospital, Merseyside, UK.

Neil Nichol
Consultant in Emergency Medicine, Ninewells Hospital, Dundee, UK.

List of contributors

Jerry Nolan
Consultant in Anaesthesia and Intensive Care, Royal United Hospital, Bath, UK.

Tim Parke
Consultant in Emergency Medicine, Southern General Hospital, Glasgow, UK.

David Ray
Consultant in Anaesthesia and Intensive Care, Royal Infirmary of Edinburgh, UK.

Neil Robinson
Consultant in Emergency Medicine, Salisbury District Hospital, Salisbury, UK.

Patricia Weir
Consultant in Paediatric Anaesthesia and Intensive Care, Bristol Royal Hospital for Children, Bristol, UK.

Dominic Williamson
Consultant in Emergency Medicine, Royal United Hospital, Bath, UK.

Paul Younge
Consultant in Emergency Medicine, Frenchay Hospital, Bristol, UK.

Foreword

This book and the course for which it is the manual are very important developments in acute patient care. Compromise of the airway or ventilation is the most urgent of all emergencies, requiring a prompt and skilled response. Being able to recognize such compromise, knowing how and when to intervene and possessing the expertise safely to do so, form a potentially life-saving combination.

Fully trained anaesthetists possess this combination, but patients with airway or ventilation problems are frequently seen by doctors who are not trained anaesthetists. It is imperative that these doctors can recognize the problem and initiate an appropriate and safe response. This book and its accompanying course are therefore designed principally for anaesthetists in the early stages of their training, and for emergency and acute physicians.

Neither this book nor the accompanying course can, by themselves, impart sufficient knowledge and skills for participants to safely manage all aspects of airway care. Both the book and the course are at pains to emphasize this. Instead they emphasize a structured approach to the problems of establishing, managing and stabilizing the airway, an excellent decision-making process, and an introduction to basic and more advanced skills in the management of the airway and ventilation. Specific chapters address key issues such as airway assessment, oxygen therapy, basic airway management techniques and indications for intubation. Rapid sequence induction, how to deal with difficult or failed intubation and post-intubation management during transfer are also all discussed in detail. In particular, the book emphasizes a team response to this most pressing of emergencies so as to ensure a safe approach, informed decision-making and the application of skills up to the limit of the practitioner's competence.

The book and the course are most appropriate for doctors in the early years of anaesthetic training or those undertaking the acute care common stem programme, but will also be of use to more senior doctors involved in acute care.

Professor Alastair McGowan OBE
Dean of Postgraduate Medicine, West of Scotland Deanery
Immediate Past President, College of Emergency medicine

Sir Peter Simpson
Immediate Past-President, Royal College of Anaesthetists

Abbreviations

ABCD	Airway, breathing, circulation and disability
ABG	Arterial blood gas
APL	Adjustable pressure limiting (valve)
APLS	Advanced paediatric life support
ARDS	Acute respiratory distress syndrome
ATLS	Advanced trauma life support
BiPAP	Bi-level positive airway pressure
BURP	Backwards, upwards, rightwards pressure
CICV	Can't intubate, can't ventilate
$CMRO_2$	Cerebral metabolic rate for oxygen
CMV	Controlled mandatory ventilation
CO_2	Carbon dioxide
COPD	Chronic obstructive pulmonary disease
CPAP	Continuous positive airway pressure
CPP	Cerebral perfusion pressure
CSI	Cervical spine injury
CT	Computed tomography
CVP	Central venous pressure
CXR	Chest X-ray
ECG	Electrocardiogram
ED	Emergency department
EEG	Electroencephalogram
ENT	Ear, nose and throat
EPAP	Expiratory positive airway pressure
$ETCO_2$	End tidal carbon dioxide
FAO_2	Fractional alveolar oxygen concentration
FG	French gauge
FGF	Fresh gas flow
FiO_2	Inspired oxygen concentration
FRC	Functional residual capacity
GABA	Gamma-amino butyric acid
GCS	Glasgow Coma Scale
GI	Gastro-intestinal
HAFOE	High-airflow oxygen enrichment
HME	Heat and moisture exchanger
ICNARC	Intensive Care National Audit And Research Centre

ICP	Intracranial pressure
ICU	Intensive care unit
I:E	Inspiratory–expiratory ratio
ILMA	Intubating laryngeal mask airway
IM	Intramuscular
IOP	Intraocular pressure
IPAP	Inspiratory positive airway pressure
IPPV	Intermittent positive pressure ventilation
IV	Intravenous
LED	Light-emitting diode
LMA	Laryngeal mask airway
MAP	Mean arterial pressure
MC	Mary Caterall
MET	Medical emergency team
MH	Malignant hyperthermia
MMC	Modernising Medical Careers
MMS	Masseter muscle spasm
MV	Minute volume
NEAR	National Emergency Airway Registry
NIBP	Non-invasive blood pressure
NICE	National Institute for Health and Clinical Excellence
NIV	Non-invasive ventilation
NMB	Neuromuscular blocker
NMJ	Neuromuscular junction
O_2	Oxygen
P_ACO_2	Partial pressure of carbon dioxide (alveolar)
P_AO_2	Partial pressure of oxygen (alveolar)
$PaCO_2$	Partial pressure of carbon dioxide (arterial)
PaO_2	Partial pressure of oxygen (arterial)
PEEP	Positive end expiratory pressure
PICU	Paediatric intensive care unit
PLMA	ProSeal laryngeal mask airway
P_{max}	Peak (maximum) inspiratory pressure
PO_2	Partial pressure of oxygen
Q	Perfusion
RR	Respiratory rate
RSI	Rapid sequence induction (of anaesthesia)
SIGN	Scottish Intercollegiate Guidelines Network
SIMV	Synchronized intermittent mandatory ventilation
SpO_2	Oxygen saturation by pulse oximetry
TBI	Traumatic brain injury

V	Ventilation
V/Q	Ventilation/perfusion ratio
VALI	Ventilator associated lung injury
V_T	Tidal volume

1

Introduction and overview

Mike Clancy, Jerry Nolan and Jonathan Benger

Objective

The objective of this chapter is:
- to understand the purpose and scope of this manual.

Introduction

Effective airway management is central to the care of critically ill and injured patients. Competency in assessment and maintenance of the airway using basic airway manoeuvres first, followed by advanced skills such as rapid sequence induction of anaesthesia and tracheal intubation, are core skills for doctors who treat seriously ill or potentially ill patients. In the UK, this typically involves the specialties of:
- anaesthesia
- emergency medicine
- intensive care medicine
- acute medicine.

The location for emergency airway management is usually outside the relatively controlled environment of an anaesthetic room, most commonly in the resuscitation room of an emergency department, but sometimes in a variety of other in-hospital and pre-hospital settings. Emergency airway management can be difficult and challenging: it requires individuals to work in relatively unfamiliar environments under conditions of stress and uncertainty, and where the principles of elective anaesthesia need modification. Information is often incomplete, normal physiology deranged, and opportunity for delay is infrequent. The problems intrinsic to these patients, such as an unstable cervical spine, poor cardiorespiratory reserve or profound metabolic dysfunction, must be anticipated and surmounted.

Emergency airway management is not simply an extension of elective anaesthesia, and specific training is essential to safely treat this challenging and heterogeneous group of patients. Individuals must practice within the limits of their own competence and work collaboratively with experienced clinicians from several disciplines to ensure patients receive optimal care (Figure 1.1).

Skills and judgement, as well as knowledge, are essential for treating patients who require emergency airway intervention. Careful judgement is required to determine whether an intervention is appropriate, how and when it should be undertaken, and what additional personnel and equipment are needed.

Emergency Airway Management, eds. Jonathan Benger, Jerry Nolan and Mike Clancy.
Published by Cambridge University Press. © College of Emergency Medicine, London 2009.

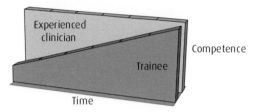

Figure 1.1 A collaborative approach ensures the best patient care.

Central to emergency airway management is the recognition of:
1 the fundamental importance of basic airways skills
2 the need for close collaboration with those who are already competent to enable effective clinical training. It is essential to work alongside practitioners who have established expertise in emergency airway care in order to build upon and apply theoretical learning. A clinician working alone should not attempt emergency airway interventions that are outside the limits of their own competence.

Audit and skills maintenance
Audit and peer review of clinical practice must be undertaken continuously to ensure standards are maintained. Further information can be found in Chapter 14. Medical simulators are becoming more sophisticated, and will have an increasing role in skill retention and assessment.

Summary
- This manual will not provide competence in emergency airway management, but offers a firm foundation upon which further training and assessment can be based.
- Effective emergency airway management requires commitment to a process of ongoing training, assessment, skill maintenance and audit that will last throughout the practitioner's professional career.

2

Delivery of oxygen

Carl Gwinnutt

Objectives

The objectives of this chapter are to:
- understand the causes of hypoxaemia
- be familiar with devices available to increase the inspired oxygen concentration
- understand the function and use of the self-inflating bag-mask
- understand the function and use of the Mapleson C breathing system
- understand how to monitor oxygenation
- understand the principle of pre-oxygenation.

Causes of hypoxaemia

The strict definition of hypoxaemia is a partial pressure of oxygen in the arterial blood (PaO_2) below normal; however, a value of <8 kPa or 60 mmHg (equivalent to an arterial oxygen saturation of approximately 90%) is often used to define hypoxaemia requiring treatment. In nearly all patients hypoxaemia can usually be improved, at least initially, by increasing the inspired oxygen concentration.

Although the cause of hypoxaemia is usually multifactorial, there are several distinct mechanisms:
- alveolar hypoventilation
- mismatch between ventilation and perfusion within the lungs
- pulmonary diffusion defects
- reduced inspired oxygen concentration.

Alveolar hypoventilation

Insufficient oxygen enters the alveoli to replace that taken up by the blood. Both the alveolar partial pressure of oxygen PAO_2 and arterial partial pressure of oxygen (PaO_2) decrease. In most patients, increasing the inspired oxygen concentration will restore alveolar and arterial PO_2. When an adult's tidal volume decreases below approximately 150 ml there is no ventilation of the alveoli, only the 'dead space', which is the volume of the airways that plays no part in gas exchange. No oxygen reaches the alveoli, irrespective of the inspired concentration, and profound hypoxaemia will follow. At this point ventilatory support and supplementary oxygen will be required. Hypoventilation is always accompanied by hypercapnia, as there is an inverse relationship between arterial partial pressure of carbon dioxide ($PaCO_2$) and alveolar ventilation.

Emergency Airway Management, eds. Jonathan Benger, Jerry Nolan and Mike Clancy.
Published by Cambridge University Press. © College of Emergency Medicine, London 2009.

Common causes of hypoventilation are as follows.

Airway obstruction:
- tongue
- blood
- vomit
- bronchospasm
- oedema (infection, burns, allergy).

Central respiratory depression:
- drugs
- alcohol
- central nervous system injury (cerebrovascular event, trauma, etc.)
- hypothermia.

Impaired mechanics of ventilation:
- pain
- pneumothorax
- haemothorax
- pulmonary oedema
- diaphragmatic splinting
- pre-existing lung disease.

Mismatch between ventilation and perfusion within the lungs

Normally, ventilation of the alveoli (V) and perfusion with blood (Q) are well matched (V/Q=1), ensuring that haemoglobin in blood leaving the lungs is saturated with oxygen (Figure 2.1). If this process is disturbed (V/Q mismatch) regions develop where:

1 perfusion exceeds ventilation (V/Q<1), resulting in haemoglobin with reduced oxygen content, e.g. pneumothorax, pneumonia

2 ventilation exceeds perfusion (V/Q>1). This can be considered wasted ventilation as very little additional oxygen is taken up when haemoglobin is already almost fully saturated (98%), e.g. hypotension.

At its most extreme, some regions of the lung may be perfused but not ventilated (V/Q=0): blood leaving these areas remains 'venous', and is often referred to as shunted blood. This is then mixed with oxygenated blood leaving ventilated regions of the lungs. The final oxygen content of blood leaving the lungs is dependent on the relative proportions of blood from these two regions:

- blood perfusing ventilated alveoli has an oxygen content of approximately 20 ml/100 ml blood (assuming a haemoglobin concentration of 15 g dl^{-1})
- blood perfusing unventilated alveoli remains 'venous', with an oxygen content of 15 ml/100 ml blood.

The effect of small regions of V/Q mismatch can be corrected by increasing the inspired oxygen concentration; however, once more than 30% of the pulmonary blood flow passes through regions where V/Q<1 hypoxaemia is inevitable, even when breathing 100% oxygen. This is because the oxygen content of the pulmonary

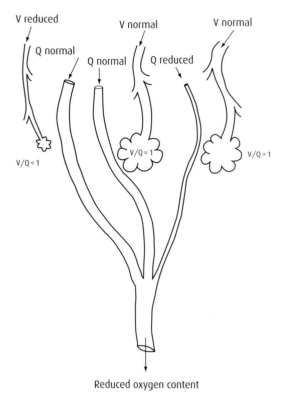

Figure 2.1 Different V/Q ratios.

blood flowing through regions ventilated with 100% oxygen will increase by only 1 ml/100 ml blood (to produce 21 ml of oxygen per 100 ml blood), and this is insufficient to offset regions of low V/Q, where the oxygen content will be only 15 ml/100 ml blood.

> For an equivalent blood flow, regions of V/Q < 1 decrease blood oxygen content more than increasing the alveolar oxygen concentration in regions of V/Q > 1

Pulmonary diffusion defects

Any chronic condition causing thickening of the alveolar membrane, e.g. fibrosing alveolitis, impairs transfer of oxygen into the blood. This is treated first by giving supplementary oxygen to increase the P_AO_2 partial pressure of oxygen in the alveoli, and then treating the underlying problem.

A reduced inspired oxygen concentration

As the inspired oxygen concentration is a prime determinant of the amount of oxygen in the alveoli, reducing this will lead to hypoxaemia. At ambient pressure there are no circumstances where it is appropriate to administer less than 21% oxygen.

Devices used for delivery of oxygen
Spontaneous ventilation

Variable-performance devices: masks or nasal cannulae These are adequate for the majority of hypoxaemic patients. The precise concentration of oxygen inspired by the patient is unknown, as it depends on the patient's respiratory pattern and the oxygen flow (usually $2–15 l\,min^{-1}$). When breathing through a mask the inspired gas consists of a mixture of:

- oxygen flowing into the mask
- oxygen that has accumulated under the mask during the expiratory pause
- alveolar gas exhaled during the previous breath that has collected under the mask
- air entrained during inspiration from the holes in the side of the mask and from leaks between the mask and face.

Examples of this type of device are Hudson and Mary Caterall (MC) masks (Figure 2.2). As a guide, they increase the inspired oxygen concentration to 25–60% with oxygen flows of $2–15 l\,min^{-1}$.

Patients unable to tolerate a facemask, but who can nose breathe, may find either a single foam tipped catheter or double catheters, placed just inside the vestibule of the nose, more comfortable (Figure 2.3). Lower flows of oxygen are used: $2–4 l\,min^{-1}$ increases the inspired oxygen concentration to 25–40%.

If higher inspired oxygen concentrations are needed in a spontaneously breathing patient, a Hudson mask with a reservoir (non-rebreathing bag) can be used (Figure 2.4). A one-way valve diverts the oxygen flow into the reservoir during expiration. During inspiration, the contents of the reservoir, along with the high flow of oxygen ($12–15 l\,min^{-1}$), ensure minimal entrainment of air, raising the inspired concentration to approximately 80%, providing that the reservoir bag inflates and deflates with each breath. This requires a well-fitting, functioning mask and reservoir, and is often overlooked in clinical practice. An inspired oxygen concentration of 100% can be achieved only by using a close-fitting facemask with an anaesthetic breathing system, combined with an oxygen flow of $12–15 l\,min^{-1}$ (see below).

Fixed-performance devices These are used when it is important to deliver a precise concentration of oxygen, unaffected by the patient's ventilatory pattern. These devices work on the principle of high-airflow oxygen enrichment (HAFOE). Oxygen is delivered to a Venturi that entrains a much greater, but constant, flow of air (Figure 2.5). The total flow into the mask may be as high as $45 l\,min^{-1}$. The high

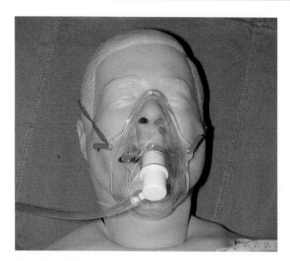

Figure 2.2 Hudson mask.

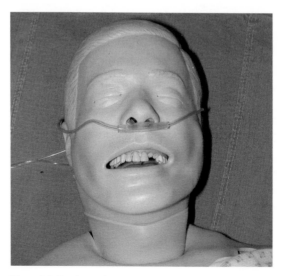

Figure 2.3 Nasal cannulae.

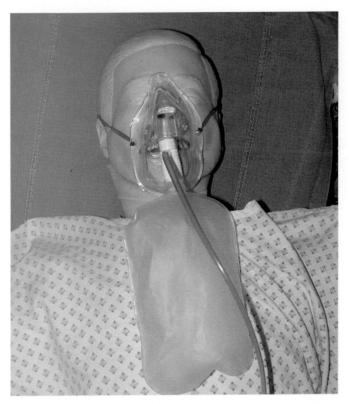

Figure 2.4 Hudson mask with reservoir.

Table 2.1. Effect of type of Venturi valve and oxygen flow on inspired oxygen concentration

Venturi valve colour	Oxygen flow rate (litres min^{-1})	Inspired oxygen concentration (%)
Blue	2	24
White	4	28
Yellow	6	35
Red	8	40
Green	12	60

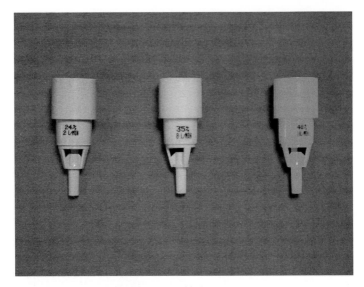

Figure 2.5 A range of Venturi devices suitable for HAFOE.

gas flow has two effects: it exceeds the patient's peak inspiratory flow, reducing entrainment of air, and flushes expiratory gas, reducing rebreathing.

These devices deliver a fixed concentration for a given flow, and there are several interchangeable Venturis to vary the oxygen concentration (Table 2.1).

The above systems all deliver dry gas to the patient, which may cause crusting or thickening of secretions, difficulty with clearance, and patient discomfort. For prolonged use, a HAFOE system should be used with a humidifier.

Assisted ventilation

Patients whose ventilation is inadequate to maintain oxygenation despite an increase in the inspired oxygen concentration using one of the devices described above, or who are apnoeic, will require oxygenation using a mechanical device. The simplest and most widely used device is the bag-mask (Figure 2.6). An alternative is an anaesthetic breathing system (Figures 2.9 and 2.10).

In selected patients improved oxygenation, as well as ventilatory assistance, can be achieved using either continuous positive airway pressure (CPAP) or bi-level positive airway pressure (BiPAP). These forms of non-invasive ventilatory support are described in Chapter 12.

The bag-mask device In its simplest form this consists of a self-inflating bag: when squeezed, the contents are delivered to the patient via a non-return valve and facemask. On release, the bag entrains air as it returns to its original shape. Expired air from the patient is prevented from reaching the bag by a one-way valve. In this manner, the patient's lungs are ventilated with air (21% oxygen). The use of modern, clear plastic facemasks has several advantages over traditional opaque masks: regurgitated stomach contents can be seen sooner, 'fogging' of the plastic during exhalation indicates that gas (oxygen) is going into and out of the lungs, and the masks are disposable, reducing the risk of cross-infection.

The oxygen concentration in the gas delivered from the bag can be increased in two ways:

1 By connecting a high flow of oxygen ($10-15 \, \mathrm{l \, min^{-1}}$) to an inlet port, usually adjacent to the air entrainment valve at the opposite end of the bag to the mask. In this way, when the bag refills, it does so with a mixture of air and oxygen. The oxygen concentration delivered to the patient will depend upon several factors including oxygen flow, rate of ventilation and volume delivered. In the average adult, the concentration is unlikely to exceed 50% (Figure 2.7).

2 In addition to the above, a reservoir can be attached over the air entrainment valve. As the bag is squeezed to ventilate the patient's lungs, the oxygen flow is diverted and accumulates within the reservoir. As the bag is released it refills from the contents of the reservoir and the oxygen flow, thereby virtually eliminating air entrainment. In this manner, providing the oxygen flow exceeds the minute ventilation of the lungs, close to 100% oxygen can be delivered (Figure 2.8).

Oxygen delivery with this device in any configuration is dependent on:

1 The practitioner being able to maintain a good seal between the facemask and the patient's face, so that there is minimal escape of gas around the mask when the bag is squeezed. This is best achieved by using a two-person technique: one holds the facemask with both hands, while the other squeezes the bag.

2 Not using high pressures to ventilate the patient's lungs. High pressures will force gas down the oesophagus and into the stomach. This will reduce ventilation of the lungs and predispose to regurgitation and aspiration.

The commonest reason for requiring high pressures to ventilate the patient's lungs is failure to maintain a patent airway. This is commonly caused by:

1 Poor airway control: this can often be overcome by using a two-person technique.

2 Foreign material in the airway, e.g. vomit, blood: this must be removed using a safe and effective suction technique.

Although a patient can breathe oxygen spontaneously from a bag-mask device, this is sub-optimal because effort is needed to overcome the resistance to inspiratory and expiratory flow. Spontaneously breathing patients should be given oxygen using one of the devices described above, or via an anaesthetic breathing system.

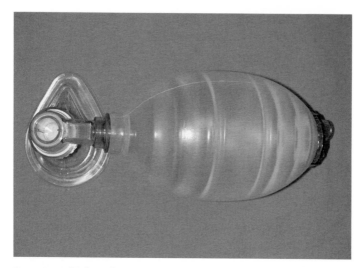

Figure 2.6 Self-inflating bag-mask.

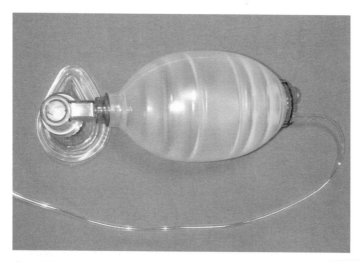

Figure 2.7 Bag-mask with oxygen attached.

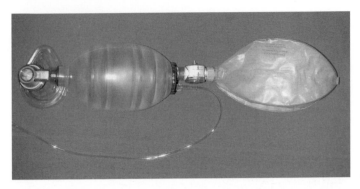

Figure 2.8 Bag-mask with oxygen and reservoir.

The anaesthetic breathing system

These are used during both spontaneous and assisted ventilation. Their safe use requires an understanding of how they function, which differs depending on whether the patient is breathing spontaneously or ventilation is assisted.

There are five basic anaesthetic breathing systems: Mapleson A, B, C, D and E. The most commonly used in emergency airway management is the Mapleson C (or Water's) breathing system; for simplicity, this is the only system that will be described in detail. Additional information can be found in the further reading section.

The Mapleson C anaesthetic system (Figures 2.9 and 2.10) comprises:

1 An oxygen input, either from the common gas outlet of an anaesthetic machine or a wall-mounted flowmeter.

2 A reservoir bag. This has several functions:

  a It collects the inflowing oxygen during expiration, which is then used to meet the patient's peak inspiratory flow during spontaneous ventilation.

  b Movement of the bag can be used as an indicator of ventilation.

  c It can be squeezed to deliver oxygen to assist ventilation.

  d If the expiratory valve is closed (or blocked) excess gas accumulates in the bag with minimal increase in airway pressure (a safety feature to protect the patient's lungs from barotrauma).

3 An adjustable, pressure limiting valve usually referred to as the expiratory (or APL) valve. This opens during expiration to enable the escape of exhaled gas (containing carbon dioxide) and prevent its accumulation within the system. This valve also enables the escape of any surplus oxygen flow. The valve can be adjusted manually from fully open (minimal opening pressure) to fully closed (no gas escape is possible through the valve).

4 A connection to a facemask: this is often a short, flexible piece of tubing that may incorporate a bacterial filter.

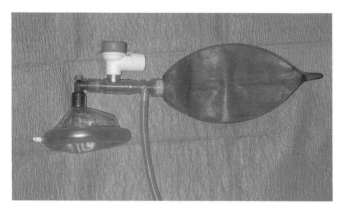

Figure 2.9 Mapleson C anaesthetic breathing system.

Mapleson C circuit (not to scale)

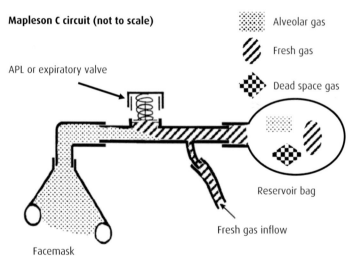

Figure 2.10 *Diagram showing functional details of the Mapleson C anaesthetic breathing system.* Diagram showing the distribution of gas in the Mapleson C circuit in a patient breathing spontaneously, immediately before inspiration. As inspiration starts the circuit delivers alveolar gas (containing CO_2), fresh gas plus a mixture from the reservoir bag. The amount of gas inspired that contains CO_2 (i.e. the degree of rebreathing) will be determined by the fresh gas flow, which has the effect of flushing CO_2 from the system.

An important feature of this system is the potential for accumulation of carbon dioxide within the reservoir bag. Although exhaled gas escapes through the expiratory valve, this will be efficiently achieved only when the oxygen flow exceeds the patient's minute volume, so that all the carbon dioxide is eliminated.

Using the Mapleson C breathing system

Spontaneous ventilation The mask is held on the patient's face with the expiratory valve fully open so that expiration is unimpeded. An oxygen flow of $12–15\,l\,min^{-1}$ is required to prevent the accumulation of carbon dioxide. As the patient breathes in, the negative pressure closes the valve and the bag will collapse slightly. During expiration the bag refills and there will be an audible leak of gas via the valve.

Assisted ventilation The mask is held on the patient's face and the expiratory valve manually adjusted (partially closed) so that sufficient pressure can be generated to inflate the lungs. The reservoir bag is squeezed (this will often require a second person) and some gas will be heard escaping via the valve. During expiration, the bag refills with oxygen and there will be an audible leak of gas via the valve. If the valve is not closed sufficiently during attempted ventilation, the oxygen escapes via the valve rather than entering the patient's lungs. Again, an oxygen flow of $12–15\,l\,min^{-1}$ will be required to prevent the accumulation of carbon dioxide.

Pitfalls when using an anaesthetic breathing system
Spontaneous ventilation
1 Inadequate oxygen flow. Carbon dioxide is not flushed from the system and accumulates in the bag. This leads to rebreathing and the patient will become hypercarbic with a range of adverse effects, e.g. increased cerebral blood flow and intracranial pressure, cardiac arrhythmias.
2 Expiratory valve closed. Insufficient venting of excess gas will cause the volume and pressure in the system to increase. This prevents expiration and also causes an increase in intrathoracic pressure that may have several serious consequences, e.g. increasing intracranial pressure, barotrauma. Gas may be forced into the stomach and predispose to regurgitation. In practice, either an increasing leak develops around the mask or the distending bag should alert the practitioner.

Assisted ventilation
1 Inadequate oxygen flow. It becomes increasingly difficult to provide adequate ventilation as the bag gradually collapses. At this point, the danger is that the expiratory valve is gradually closed to prevent escape of gas and maintain enough volume in the system to squeeze the bag. Although this will enable the patient's lungs to be ventilated, carbon dioxide is not eliminated and accumulates within the system. The patient becomes rapidly hypercarbic with the problems described above.

Because of the specialist nature of anaesthetic breathing systems, only those with appropriate training should use them.

Monitoring oxygenation
The pulse oximeter

A probe, containing a light-emitting diode (LED) and a photodetector, is applied across the tip of a digit or earlobe. The LED emits red light alternately at two different wavelengths, in the visible and infrared regions of the electromagnetic spectrum. These are transmitted through the tissues and absorbed to different degrees by oxyhaemoglobin and deoxyhaemoglobin. The intensity of light reaching the photodetector is converted to an electrical signal. The absorption by the tissues and venous blood is static. This is then subtracted from the beat-to-beat variation in absorption due to arterial blood to display the peripheral arterial oxygen saturation (SpO_2), both as a waveform and a digital reading. Pulse oximeters are accurate to $\pm 2\%$. The waveform can also indicate the heart rate. Alarms are provided for arterial blood saturation and heart rate values. The pulse oximeter therefore gives information about both the circulatory and respiratory systems, and has the advantages of:

- providing continuous monitoring of oxygenation at tissue level
- being unaffected by skin pigmentation
- portability (mains or battery powered)
- non-invasive.

  There are several important limitations to this device:

- failure to realize the severity of hypoxaemia: because of the shape of the oxyhaemoglobin dissociation curve (Figure 2.12), a saturation of 90% equates to a PaO_2 of 8 kPa (60 mmHg)
- unreliability when there is severe vasoconstriction, because of the reduced pulsatile component of the signal
- provides no indication of the $PaCO_2$: profound hypercapnia is possible with normal oxygen saturations, particularly in the presence of alveolar hypoventilation and a high concentration of inspired oxygen
- unreliable with certain haemoglobins:
  a when carboxyhaemoglobin is present, it overestimates SaO_2
  b when methaemoglobin is present, at saturations greater than 85% it underestimates SaO_2
- progressively under-reads the saturation as the haemoglobin decreases (but is not affected by polycythaemia)
- affected by extraneous light
- unreliable when there is excessive movement of the patient.

The pulse oximeter is not an indicator of the adequacy of alveolar ventilation

Arterial blood gas analysis

The analysis of an arterial blood gas sample is essential for assessing the adequacy of oxygenation and ventilation. Information on the interpretation of arterial blood gases can be found in the further reading section.

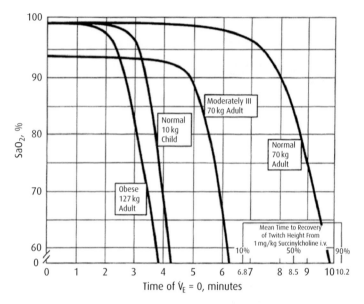

Figure 2.11 *Time to desaturation according to a range of patient characteristics.*
Time to haemoglobin desaturation with initial $FAO_2 = 0.87$ for various patient
circumstances. Note the bars indicating recovery from succinylcholine paralysis at
the bottom right of the graph. (From Benumof, J., Dagg, R. & Benumof, R. (1997)
Critical hemoglobin desaturation will occur before return to an unparalyzed
state following 1 mg/kg intravenous succinylcholine. *Anesthesiology*; **87**: 979–82,
with permission.)

Pre-oxygenation

Effective pre-oxygenation enables several minutes of apnoea, without desaturation of arterial blood, during which tracheal intubation can be achieved.
An oxygen reservoir is developed by replacing air in the lungs (the functional
residual capacity) with oxygen, and saturating the blood and tissues. The most
efficient way of achieving this is by giving 100% oxygen via a Mapleson
C breathing system. A bag-mask device is a less suitable alternative because of
the resistance to inspiratory and expiratory flow, and inability to deliver 100%
oxygen. An oxygen mask with a properly functioning reservoir bag delivers
approximately 80% oxygen and is an alternative, although less effective, method
if an anaesthetic breathing system is not immediately available, or the patient
will not tolerate a tightly fitting facemask.

The time for arterial blood to desaturate is related to the effectiveness of
the pre-oxygenation phase, the age and weight of the patient, and the patient's

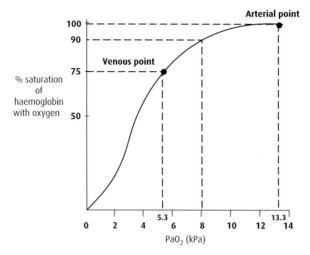

Figure 2.12 *The oxygen–haemoglobin dissociation curve.* The shape of the oxygen–haemoglobin dissociation curve indicates that the oxygen saturation of blood decreases rapidly below 92%; therefore, when the oxygen saturation displayed on the pulse oximeter decreases to 92% corrective action is required, and the patient should be re-oxygenated immediately.

physiological status. In a healthy adult following effective pre-oxygenation, the time for arterial blood to desaturate to 92% may be as much as eight minutes; for a child, this is reduced to four minutes. All these times are reduced in an ill patient, who is usually unable to achieve full pre-oxygenation, especially if ventilation is inadequate (Figure 2.11). Once the saturation reaches 92%, the rate of desaturation accelerates because of the shape of the oxyhaemoglobin dissociation curve (Figure 2.12).

Summary
- The commonest causes of hypoxaemia are hypoventilation and ventilation/perfusion mismatch, both of which can be initially managed by increasing the inspired oxygen concentration.
- A variety of devices are available to deliver oxygen in patients breathing spontaneously or requiring assisted ventilation.
- The pulse oximeter provides a useful indication of arterial oxygenation, but not the adequacy of ventilation.
- Pre-oxygenation is an important step in preparing for rapid sequence induction, and is best achieved using an anaesthetic breathing system.

Further reading

1 West, J.B. (2004) *Respiratory Physiology – The Essentials*, 7th edn. Philadelphia: Lippincott, Williams and Wilkins.

2 Nolan, J., Soar, J., Lockey, A. *et al.* eds. (2006) *Advanced Life Support*, 5th edn. London: Resuscitation Council.

3 Leach, R.M. & Bateman, N.T. (1993) Acute oxygen therapy. *Br J Hosp Med*; **49**: 637–44.

4 Gwinnutt, C.L. (1996) *Clinical Anaesthesia*. Oxford: Blackwell Science.

5 Driscoll, P., Brown, T., Gwinnutt, C. & Wardle, T. (1997) *A Simple Guide to Blood Gas Analysis*. London: BMJ Publishing Group.

Airway assessment

Dominic Williamson and Jerry Nolan

Objectives

The objectives of this chapter are to:

- discuss the rationale for airway assessment
- outline a pre-anaesthetic patient assessment
- evaluate methods of airway assessment
- identify patients who may be difficult to ventilate and/or intubate
- identify patients that may require a different airway intervention.

Introduction

During elective anaesthesia a failed airway ('can't intubate, can't ventilate') occurs in 0.01–0.03% of cases. Difficult intubation, defined as the need for more than three attempts, occurs in 1.15–3.8% of elective surgical cases, and is usually related to a poor view at laryngoscopy. However, the characteristics of patients requiring intubation or assisted ventilation outside the operating theatre are different to those undergoing elective surgical procedures, and the incidence of difficult intubation is significantly higher in emergency departments. More importantly, a failed airway may occur at least ten times more frequently in the emergency setting: in the United States, 0.5% of intubations recorded in the National Emergency Airway Registry (NEAR) required a surgical airway. In a recent Scottish study, 57/671 (8.5%) of patients undergoing rapid sequence induction in the emergency department had Cormack and Lehane grade 3 or 4 views at laryngoscopy (see below), and two (0.3%) required a surgical airway.

Given these data, difficulties with the airway must be expected in all emergency patients, and appropriate preparation undertaken. Some features may indicate a particularly high likelihood of airway difficulties, and in these cases modification of practice may reduce complications and improve outcome.

Definition of a difficult airway

A difficult airway is categorized by the following.

Difficult mask ventilation

Difficult mask ventilation occurs when the patient's anatomy or injuries make it impossible to maintain adequate ventilation and oxygenation with a facemask and simple airway adjuncts alone.

Emergency Airway Management, eds. Jonathan Benger, Jerry Nolan and Mike Clancy.
Published by Cambridge University Press. © College of Emergency Medicine, London 2009.

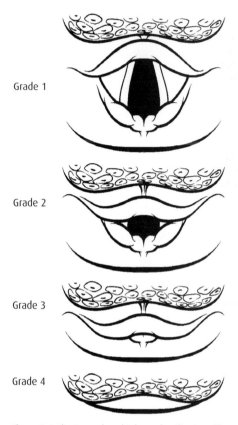

Figure 3.1 The Cormack and Lehane classification of laryngeal view: *Grade 1* The vocal cords are visible; *Grade 2* The vocals cords are only partly visible; *Grade 3* Only the epiglottis is seen; *Grade 4* The epiglottis cannot be seen.

Difficult view at laryngoscopy

The view at laryngoscopy has been classified by Cormack and Lehane (Figure 3.1). A difficult view is defined as being unable to see any portion of the vocal cords with conventional laryngoscopy (Cormack and Lehane grades 3 and 4). These views are associated with more difficult or even impossible intubations under direct vision. Although this may not help at initial presentation, the grade of view at laryngoscopy must be recorded because it may influence the approach to future airway management by other healthcare professionals.

Difficult intubation

Difficult intubation has been defined as occurring when an experienced laryngoscopist, using direct laryngoscopy, requires:

1 more than two attempts with the same blade or;
2 a change in the blade or an adjunct to a direct laryngoscope (e.g. bougie) or;
3 use of an alternative device or technique following failed intubation with direct laryngoscopy.

Difficult cricothyroidotomy

Failure to intubate the trachea combined with an inability to ventilate the patient's lungs, using a bag-mask or laryngeal mask airway (LMA), will necessitate a surgical airway. Very rarely, the patient's cricothyroid membrane is inaccessible. This makes induction of anaesthesia particularly risky because if the airway is lost it may be irretrievable.

General assessment of patients before inducing anaesthesia

Few patients require immediate induction of anaesthesia and intubation. Some time is usually available for formal assessment, and in almost all cases a comprehensive evaluation of the patient is required before inducing anaesthesia (see Box 3.1).

Box 3.1 Pre-anaesthetic assessment of emergency patients where time allows

- comprehensive history
- cardiorespiratory status
- conscious level
- focal/global neurological signs
- assessment of face and neck
- assessment for pneumothorax
- abdominal and pelvic assessment for surgical signs
- body morphology.

When time allows, obtain a good history including current medication and allergies, previous medical and surgical problems, last oral intake, and details of the patient's current condition. If available, previous medical records can be invaluable. Patients and relatives may have been informed about any serious problems, including airway difficulties, occurring during previous anaesthetics. A MedicAlert bracelet system has been advocated for patients with difficult airways, and may be carried by some.

All pre-anaesthetic findings must be documented clearly and handed over to the team responsible for the patient's continuing care.

Once a patient is anaesthetized some physical signs will be lost, e.g. abdominal guarding. Before inducing anaesthesia particular attention should be paid to:

- the Glasgow Coma Scale (GCS)
- focal neurological signs
- evidence of pathology in the chest, abdomen or pelvis.

Positive pressure ventilation may convert a simple pneumothorax into a tension pneumothorax. The presence of a pneumothorax must be considered and sought by clinical examination. A chest X-ray taken before induction of anaesthesia should be considered in patients at particular risk, e.g. trauma, asthma and chronic obstructive pulmonary disease (COPD). A pneumothorax will sometimes require drainage before or immediately after induction of anaesthesia.

Intravenous anaesthetics are cardiovascular depressants and these effects will be compounded by positive pressure ventilation. Concurrent rapid infusion of intravenous fluid, combined with a vasopressor if necessary, will reduce the risk of cardiovascular collapse during induction of anaesthesia.

Airway assessment
Predicting difficulty in bag-mask ventilation

If intubation is difficult or impossible, ventilation of the patient's lungs with a bag-mask will maintain oxygenation until the airway is secured. Difficulty with facemask ventilation is a serious problem, and every effort should be made to anticipate this complication. In many cases, difficulty with facemask ventilation may be resolved by simple airway manoeuvres, and if these fail insertion of a laryngeal mask airway. This will enable oxygenation and ventilation until a definitive airway is established.

Difficult facemask ventilation will occur if it is not possible to establish a good seal, if airway patency is difficult to maintain, or if airway resistance is high or lung and chest wall compliance is poor. A study of patients undergoing elective surgery identified five criteria that were independent predictors of difficult mask ventilation: age >55 years, body mass index $>26 \mathrm{kg} \, \mathrm{m}^{-2}$, beard, lack of teeth and a history of snoring.

Features likely to cause difficulty in achieving a good seal with a facemask

- dysmorphic or asymmetrical facial features
- a beard or moustache. This can often be rectified by the application of petroleum jelly or aqueous lubricant
- significant cachexia, missing molar teeth or missing dentures causing sunken cheeks. Where possible, well-fitting dentures should be left in place. When this is not feasible the cheeks may be padded out with dressing gauze or similar
- facial trauma, particularly lacerations through the cheek and unstable bony injuries.

Features likely to cause difficulty in maintaining
an airway without intubation
- immobilized neck
- unstable facial bony injuries
- upper airway obstruction, e.g. blood or vomit, retropharyngeal swelling such as haematoma or infection
- obesity
- macroglossia
- history of snoring.

Features likely to make it difficult to ventilate the lungs
- abdominal distension/diaphragmatic splinting
- lower airways obstruction, e.g. asthma, pneumothorax
- obesity.

Predicting difficult intubation

Most tests used to predict difficult intubation have poor sensitivity and specificity. That is to say if the test is positive it does not necessarily follow that the patient will be difficult to intubate, and if negative it does not rule out the possibility of a difficult intubation. Features that have some value in predicting difficult intubation include the following.

Previous history of a difficult airway
- Look for a MedicAlert bracelet or similar. Ask about previous anaesthetic events.

Body morphology
- Morbid obesity is an independent predictor of a difficult airway.

Facial features
- Poor mouth opening – less than 4–5 cm or three finger breadths incisor to incisor (or gum to gum in edentulous patients) – will reduce access and view of the larynx.
- Prominent upper incisors will restrict view and access. Jagged teeth may puncture the cuff of a tracheal tube.
- A high arched palate reduces the space inside the mouth, compromising access during laryngoscopy.
- Receding mandible (see thyromental distance below).
- An inability to move the lower teeth in front of the upper teeth (prognath) may indicate an immobile mandible, which could restrict the view at laryngoscopy.
- Macroglossia reduces space within the mouth and makes the tongue harder to move.
- Facial trauma causing deranged facial anatomy. Bleeding into the soft tissues may distort the anatomy and normal colouration of the pharynx and larynx, making landmarks more difficult to identify. Fractures involving the temporomandibular

joints may be particularly dangerous as they can prevent any mouth opening even after a neuromuscular blocker has been given. Paradoxically, unstable, and therefore mobile, facial bony injuries may facilitate laryngoscopy and subsequent intubation.

Neck
- Thyromental distance <6–7 cm, or four finger breadths, from the top of the thyroid cartilage to the anterior border of the mandible with the head in full extension on the neck implies a short mandible and/or a high larynx: both may impair the view at laryngoscopy or make intubation very difficult.
- Trauma. Blunt trauma may rarely fracture the larynx, altering the anatomy and making it difficult to identify structures during laryngoscopy.
- Penetrating trauma may cause haematomas that displace the larynx, making the view and access difficult, yet are not visible externally.
- Infection causing either generalized swelling (e.g. pharyngitis, laryngitis, epi-glottitis) or focal swelling (retropharyngeal abscess or quinsy) may cause obstruction.
- Tumour or previous surgery.
- Reduced neck mobility will worsen the view of the larynx. The best views are obtained in adults with the head in extension and the neck in flexion. This is the 'sniffing the morning air' position, which aligns the airway axes and makes it easier to see the glottis (see Chapter 4). Reduced neck mobility may be present in presumed or actual cervical spine injury, the elderly, in patients with arthritis of the cervical spine, and in patients with previous neck injuries or surgery. During laryngoscopy with in-line stabilization of the neck and pressure applied to the cricoid cartilage the view of the glottis will be Cormack and Lehane grade 3 or 4 in 20% of cases. In obese patients, women with large breasts, or patients with severe fixed flexion neck deformities (e.g. ankylosing spondylitis), it may even be difficult to get the laryngoscope blade into the mouth whilst mounted on the handle. In these cases the blade may have to be inserted separately or a specialist laryngo-scope used (such as a polio blade or a fibre optic scope).

The Mallampati score A score of I to IV is used to describe the view of the patient's tongue, faucial pillars, uvula and posterior pharynx (Figure 3.2). To be valid, the assessment is undertaken with the patient seated in front of the practitioner, and therefore has a very limited role in the assessment of patients requiring emergency airway management.

Predicting a difficult cricothyroidotomy
Performing a surgical or needle cricothyroidotomy is a rescue procedure that may enable oxygenation of a patient in a 'can't intubate, can't ventilate' scenario. These techniques rely on the cricothyroid membrane being accessible, which may not always be the case.

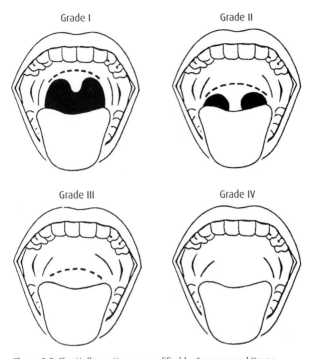

Grade I Grade II

Grade III Grade IV

Figure 3.2 The Mallampati score, modified by Samsoon and Young.

Features that may cause difficulty in accessing the cricothyroid membrane

- Obesity. A layer of subcutaneous tissues makes the anatomical landmarks ill defined and difficult to locate.
- Neck immobility. Being unable to extend the head on the neck may restrict access, particularly in the obese or short-necked patient.
- Local trauma. Significant blunt or penetrating trauma may distort the anatomy.

HAVNOT

A simple reminder for assessing predictors of a difficult airway is:

H History – including previous airway problems

A Anatomy – features of the face, mouth and teeth that may suggest intubation will be difficult

V Visual clues – obesity, facial hair, age

N Neck mobility and accessibility, including the presence of in-line stabilization

O Opening of the mouth – less than three fingers' breadth suggests potential difficulty with intubation

T Trauma – the possibility of anatomical disruption and blood in the airway.

What to do if a difficult airway is predicted

If a difficult airway is predicted, a rapid sequence induction should not be undertaken in the absence of the most experienced available assistance unless the patient has life-threatening hypoxaemia and is deteriorating despite all possible basic airway interventions. The management of a difficult and failed airway is described in more detail in Chapter 9.

Summary

- Always be prepared for a difficult airway.
- No single airway assessment tool is sufficiently sensitive or specific to reliably predict or rule out a difficult airway.
- In many cases features of the patient's morphology and pathology enable prediction of a difficult airway.
- Rarely, patients with no predictive features may be difficult or impossible to intubate using conventional techniques.
- Intubation is rarely so urgent that airway assessment is not possible: aim to undertake a pre-anaesthetic assessment in all but the most unusual cases, and document the findings.

Further reading

1 Crosby, E.T., Cooper, R.M., Douglas, M.J. *et al.* (1998) The unanticipated difficult airway with recommendations for management. *Can J Anaesth*; **45**: 757–76.

2 Cormack R.S. & Lehane, J. (1984) Difficult tracheal intubation in obstetrics. *Anaesthesia*; **39**: 1105–11.

3 Bair, A.E., Filbin, M.R., Kulkarni, R.G. & Walls, R.M. (2002) The failed intubation attempt in the emergency department: analysis of prevalence, rescue techniques, and personnel. *J Emerg Med*; **23**: 131–40.

4 Graham, C.A., Beard, D., Oglesby, A.J. *et al.* (2003) Rapid sequence intubation in Scottish urban emergency departments. *Emerg Med J*; **20**: 3–5.

5 Langeron, O., Masso, E., Huraux, C. *et al.* (2000) Prediction of difficult mask ventilation. *Anesthesiology*; **92**: 1229–35.

6 El Ganzouri, A.R., McCarthy, R.J., Tuman, K.J., Tanck, E.N. & Ivankovich, A.D. (1996) Preoperative airway assessment: predictive value of a multivariate risk index. *Anesth Analg*; **82**: 1197–204.

7 Nolan, J.P. & Wilson, M.E. (1993) Orotracheal intubation in patients with potential cervical spine injuries. An indication for the gum elastic bougie. *Anaesthesia*; **48**: 630–3.

8 Mallampati, S.R., Gatt, S.P., Gugino, L.D. *et al.* (1985) A clinical sign to predict difficult tracheal intubation: a prospective study. *Can Anaesth Soc J*; **32**: 429–34.

9 Samsoon, G.L.T. & Young, J.R.B. (1987) Difficult tracheal intubation: a retrospective study. *Anaesthesia*; **42**: 487–90.

4

Basic airway management techniques

Stephen Bush and David Ray

Objectives

The objectives of this chapter are to:

- understand the importance of basic airway management in relation to advanced airway skills
- be familiar with basic airway management techniques.

Introduction

> Basic airway management is the foundation upon which advanced airway skills are based

Basic airway manoeuvres, although apparently simple, may be both difficult and life-saving. Basic airway management is a vital component of any airway intervention: there is little point acquiring expertise in advanced techniques if the practitioner cannot open the airway and ventilate the patient's lungs.

Airway obstruction can occur at any level from the mouth to the carina. Posterior tongue displacement, blood, secretions, teeth, vomit and foreign bodies are common causes. Oedema and direct airway injury are comparatively rare causes of airway obstruction. In most patients, a combination of positioning, airway manoeuvres, adjuncts and assisted ventilation will enable sufficient oxygenation to maintain life. These interventions are considered below.

Positioning

To optimize air-flow the head, neck and torso must be positioned to align the oral, pharyngeal and laryngeal axes. Figure 4.1 shows the sub-optimal C-shaped alignment of the airway axes when the adult head and neck are in the neutral position.

In an adult patient the airway axes are better aligned when the neck is flexed on the torso and the head is extended on the neck: the so-called 'sniffing the morning air' position (Figure 4.2).

This position is easily achieved by placing a pillow or folded blanket under the patient's head. This flexes the neck on the torso, the thickness of the support determining the amount of neck flexion. Once this is maintained satisfactorily, the practitioner may gently extend the head on the neck to align the three airway axes.

Emergency Airway Management, eds. Jonathan Benger, Jerry Nolan and Mike Clancy.
Published by Cambridge University Press. © College of Emergency Medicine, London 2009.

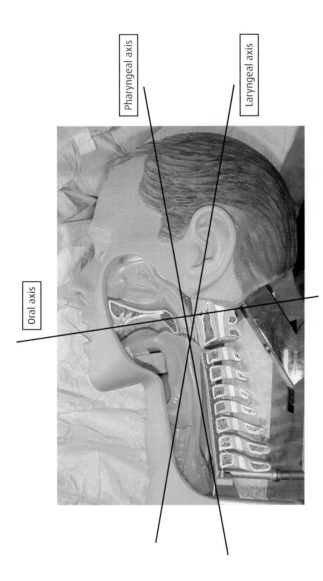

Oral axis

Pharyngeal axis

Laryngeal axis

Figure 4.1 The C-shaped curve that is formed between the oral axis, pharyngeal axis and laryngeal axis when the head and neck are in the neutral position.

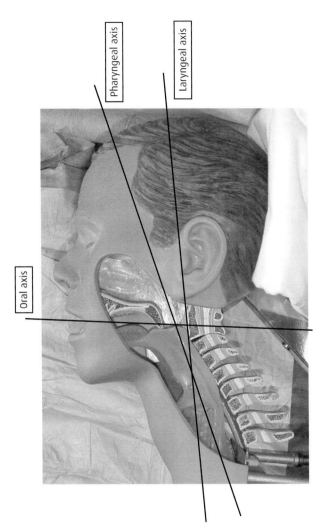

Pharyngeal axis

Laryngeal axis

Oral axis

Figure 4.2 Aligning the oral axis, pharyngeal axis and laryngeal axis by flexing the neck and extending the head.

It is important not to force the head and neck into this position in elderly patients or those with kyphosis or limited neck movement.

If a cervical spine injury is suspected the neck must be maintained in a neutral position

If the head cannot be positioned optimally, e.g. when cervical stabilization is required after trauma, backwards upwards and rightwards laryngeal pressure (the BURP manoeuvre) may help to align the axes. This is illustrated in Figure 4.3, and described in more detail in Chapter 7.

The most frequent positioning error is a progressive hyperextension of the head and neck: if head support is not used the neck is extended instead of being flexed, and the airway is occluded (Figure 4.4).

Positioning of the patient is even more important if the airway is predicted to be difficult. In some cases flexion of the neck on a pillow may not achieve the best position. In obese patients, and others who have relatively short necks, standard neck positioning may flex the head, forcing the chin onto the chest wall. This impedes access to the neck and may prevent the laryngoscope blade from entering the mouth because the anterior chest wall or the hand of an assistant applying cricoid pressure obstructs the handle. The key to correct positioning of the obese patient is to make sure that the chin is higher than the highest point of the chest or abdomen. This can often be achieved by placing one pillow under the shoulders and raising the head further using additional pillows. Figures 4.5 and 4.6 demonstrate the effect of placing the head on a single pillow, and the use of additional pillows to support the shoulders and neck, thereby permitting increased neck flexion and head extension with better alignment of the airway axes, as well as making it easier for the laryngoscope blade to enter the mouth. Raising the head end of the trolley or bed also improves pre-oxygenation in obese patients by reducing the pressure of the abdominal contents on the diaphragm, thereby increasing the functional residual capacity. Often optimal positioning is best determined from the side rather than from the head of the patient.

These principles of positioning apply equally to basic airway interventions and to the more advanced airway skills of laryngoscopy and tracheal intubation (see Chapter 6).

Airway manoeuvres

Once the airway is positioned, two other movements may further improve the airway: chin lift and jaw thrust.

Chin lift

Chin lift opens the airway by pulling the mandible forward and lifting the tongue off the posterior pharyngeal wall. The practitioner places the fingers of one hand under the mandible and lifts gently upwards (Figure 4.7). The thumb of the same hand

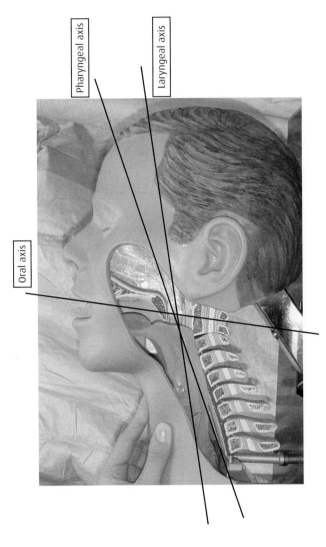

Oral axis

Pharyngeal axis

Laryngeal axis

Figure 4.3 Improvement in the alignment of the oral axis, pharyngeal axis and laryngeal axis with the BURP manoeuvre (backwards, upwards and rightwards laryngeal pressure).

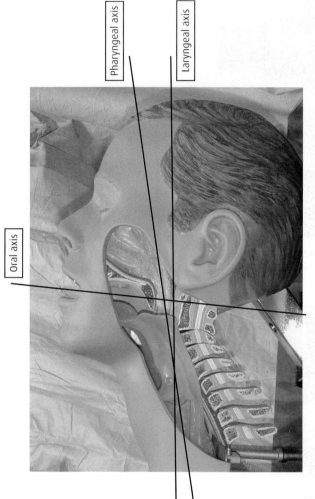

Figure 4.4 The effect of neck hyperextension on the alignment of the oral axis, pharyngeal axis and laryngeal axis.

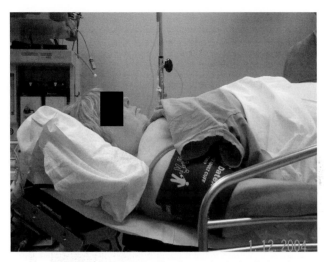

Figure 4.5 The effect of placing a single pillow under the head of an obese patient: note head flexion, with the chin impinging on the chest.

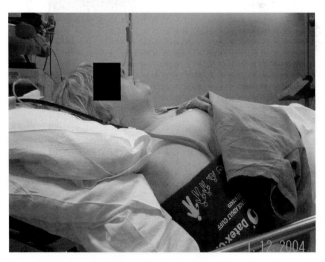

Figure 4.6 The use of additional pillows to increase neck flexion and head extension, improving alignment of the airway axes.

can be used to depress the lower lip, thereby opening the mouth. The chin lift cannot be used easily at the same time as holding a facemask over the patient's face, as the practitioner's thumb obstructs the correct positioning of the facemask. It may also become uncomfortable for the practitioner to maintain this manoeuvre for a long time.

Jaw thrust

The jaw thrust manoeuvre enables the simultaneous application of a facemask. In this technique, the practitioner's fingers are placed under and behind the angles of the mandible. The thumbs may be placed as for the chin lift, to open the mouth, or used together with the index fingers to hold a mask onto the patient's face. The mandible is then lifted forwards and upwards, lifting the tongue off the posterior pharyngeal wall (Figure 4.8).

If these manoeuvres improve the airway significantly then better oxygenation may improve the patient's conscious level.

Suction

Suction is essential for removing any liquid in the upper airway. The sucker is not used as a diagnostic tool to see if liquid is present: it must be used gently, under direct vision. Advancing the tip blindly may cause airway trauma, vagal stimulation, increased intracranial pressure and vomiting. To avoid mucosal occlusion of the sucker tip an intermediate setting should be used initially, and then adjusted as required.

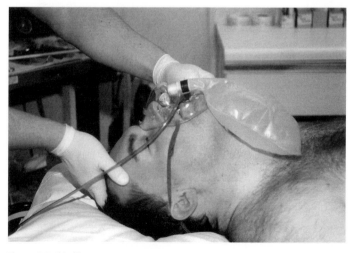

Figure 4.7 Chin lift.

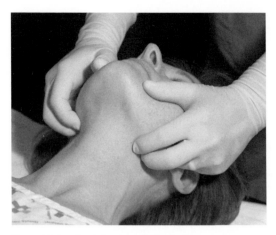

Figure 4.8 Jaw thrust. Courtesy of Mike Scott.

Airway adjuncts

If a manual manoeuvre is needed to open the airway an adjunct such as an oropharyngeal or nasopharyngeal airway will often enhance both ventilation and practitioner comfort, particularly if assisted ventilation is not required immediately, and the practitioner is not required to hold the facemask firmly on the patient's face. These devices enable the airway to be supported without the need for application of force by the practitioner.

Oropharyngeal airways

Oropharyngeal airways are hard plastic devices that are shaped to follow the contours of the oropharynx. They are manufactured in various colours and materials but share the same overall design, consisting of a flange and body comprising straight and curved components (Figure 4.9). They have a lumen to maintain airway patency and enable passage of a suction catheter to clear the oropharynx. Their shape lifts the tongue off the posterior pharyngeal wall, and the wide lumen presents little resistance to air flow.

Indications The primary indication for oropharyngeal airway insertion is an obstructed airway, or an airway that requires active manoeuvres for maintenance. These devices should be used only in patients with obtunded cough and gag reflexes (see below).

Sizing The airway is sized by placing it on the patient's face and measuring its length along a vertical line from the patient's incisors to the angle of the jaw. Correct sizing is important to reduce the likelihood of obstruction.

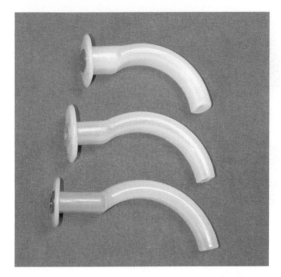

Figure 4.9 Oropharyngeal airways.

Insertion The airway is inserted upside down into the mouth. Once the tip has passed the hard palate the airway is rotated 180 degrees and advanced over the tongue. An alternative method is to use a tongue depressor or a laryngoscope blade to depress the tongue and then insert the airway the correct way up under direct vision.

Complications Insertion of an oropharyngeal airway in a patient who retains some airway reflexes may cause gagging, laryngospasm, vomiting, raised intracranial pressure and predispose to aspiration of gastric or oropharyngeal contents.

Limitations As a general guide, a patient who tolerates an oropharyngeal airway has impaired airway protective reflexes indicating the need for placement of a definitive airway. The oropharyngeal airway maintains, but does not protect, the airway; however, it will enable oxygenation before tracheal intubation. Should the increase in oxygenation improve the conscious level then intubation may not be necessary. If this occurs, or if the patient's conscious level improves for any other reason, the oral airway may need to be removed.

A patient with an oral airway must not be left unattended

Nasopharyngeal airways
Nasopharyngeal airways are soft, curved tubes with a bevel at one end and a flange at the other (Figure 4.10). Like oropharyngeal airways, they are

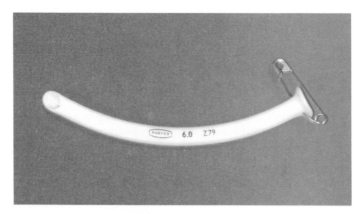

Figure 4.10 Nasopharyngeal airway.

manufactured in various colours and materials but share the same overall design. Some airways are supplied with safety pins to avoid displacement into the nostril: the safety pin should be placed through the flange of the device before the airway is inserted.

Indications Nasopharyngeal airways improve the airway by splinting open the posterior nasopharynx. Their great advantage over oropharyngeal airways is that they may be inserted in patients with intact airway reflexes without the significant risk of gagging, vomiting or aspiration associated with oral devices. They are also very useful in patients with limited mouth opening.

Sizing The traditional methods for sizing a nasopharyngeal airway (measurement against the patient's little finger or anterior nares) do not correlate with airway anatomy, and are unreliable. An appropriate size of airway in adults is 6 mm internal diameter for an average female and 7 mm internal diameter for an average male. If the airway is too long it may stimulate airway reflexes and induce vomiting. If too short, the tip may become occluded by the nasal mucosa.

Insertion The technique of insertion is simple and must be gentle. Select the nostril that appears larger and less obstructed by the nasal septum. The airway and the nostril should both be well lubricated with a water-based gel. The tip of the airway is inserted into the nostril and directed posteriorly along the transverse floor of the nose. Slight rotation of the airway during insertion may be helpful.

If insertion of a nasopharyngeal airway into a nostril is difficult, it is usually easier (and safer) to use the other nostril

Some resistance is often felt as the airway passes the turbinates, but if this is significant a smaller airway should be selected to minimize complications. Insertion of a second airway into the other nostril may improve air flow further.

Complications Nasopharyngeal airways may cause profuse haemorrhage: use of a vasoconstrictor spray before insertion may reduce the risk of bleeding.

Limitations Relative contraindications to nasopharyngeal airway insertion include basal skull fracture or significant facial injury with damage to the cribriform plate. The presence of these injuries may result in intracranial placement of the airway; however, this complication is unlikely and in the presence of life-threatening hypoxaemia and where insertion of an oropharyngeal airway is not possible, gentle and careful insertion of a nasopharyngeal airway using the above technique may be life-saving.

> The effectiveness of any airway manoeuvre or adjunct must always be assessed after it has been completed

Oxygenation
Spontaneous ventilation
Methods of oxygen delivery to a spontaneously breathing patient are described in Chapter 2.

Assisted ventilation
Even if spontaneous ventilatory efforts are present, they may be inadequate for effective gas exchange. The frequency of these efforts and the adequacy of tidal volume should be assessed by examining chest movement. Arterial blood gas analysis is helpful in the assessment of whether assisted ventilation is needed.

Should assisted ventilation be needed, the usual first step is a bag-mask technique. Although apparently simple, effective bag-mask ventilation requires several potentially difficult manoeuvres to be performed well.

Mask application The correct size of mask must be used. This is one that covers the face from the nasal bridge to the alveolar ridge. Transparent masks are recommended to enable observation of the inner surface for 'fogging' or vomiting. Some slight movement of the mask on the face is usually required for an optimal seal. Hold the mask on the face with the thumb and index finger after gently opening the airway. Spread the other fingers out along the lower border of the mandible and, ideally, place the little finger behind the angle of the mandible. These three fingers should pull the mandible up to the mask, rather than the mask being pushed down onto the mandible. Insertion of an oropharyngeal and/or nasopharyngeal airway may assist in maintaining the airway. In the unconscious or obtunded patient the jaw thrust manoeuvre is very useful when used in conjunction with application of the facemask.

Sealing techniques A poor mask seal may occur if the patient has a beard, is edentulous or is emaciated. The use of a water-based gel, leaving well-fitting dentures in place, or packing the cheeks with gauze rolls may improve the seal. A poor seal will lead to an air leak and cause poor ventilation.

Choice of equipment Most practitioners are familiar with the self-inflating bag. This device comprises a thick-walled ventilation bag, a reservoir, and a one-way valve that prevents subsequent inspiration of expired gas. The valve mechanism can become stuck if blocked by secretions, blood or vomit. Most self-inflating bags are now single use only, but if a reusable bag is used a breathing filter is attached before use. The self-inflating bag re-expands after compression even without gas flow, and therefore enables ventilation to continue in the event of a gas supply failure. For this reason a self-inflating bag and mask must accompany patients who require, or may require, assisted ventilation during all transfers.

Although the self-inflating bag is an excellent device for assisted ventilation, the one-way valve causes some resistance to gas flow in spontaneous ventilation. If the patient is breathing adequately, supplemental oxygen is best provided by other means (see Chapter 2).

> A self-inflating bag and mask must accompany the transfer of any patient who may require assisted ventilation

Ventilation Effective assisted ventilation requires a good mask seal to minimize leakage. Avoid high airway pressures; this reduces the possibility of gastric inflation, with subsequent regurgitation and aspiration. Cricoid pressure may be applied to reduce this risk, but is difficult to maintain for a long time. Partial airway obstruction can cause high airway pressures; therefore a two-person technique is recommended, especially for inexperienced practitioners. This technique enables one practitioner to use both hands to open the airway and hold the mask firmly on the face whilst a second practitioner compresses the bag. The practitioner opening the airway has both hands available for the task, and is likely to be much more effective.

If the airway pressure remains high while using the two-person technique, insertion of a nasopharyngeal airway into each nostril and an oropharyngeal airway into the oropharynx may be helpful. Use suction to remove any foreign material in the airway, and ensure the patient is correctly positioned.

> The first solution for failed bag-mask ventilation is better bag-mask ventilation!

If the patient is making some respiratory effort, the assisted ventilations should be synchronized with the patient's own efforts. Poor synchronization will cause high airway pressures, inadequate ventilation and subsequent gastric inflation with potential aspiration.

Summary
- Basic airway management is the foundation upon which advanced airway skills are based.
- Correct positioning of the head and neck is essential to ensure the best airway, but care must be taken in suspected cervical spine injury.
- Airway manoeuvres may also be needed to open the airway.
- Airway adjuncts such as oro- and nasopharyngeal airways are useful in supporting the airway.
- Assisted ventilation is required when respiratory efforts are inadequate; this may be achieved with a bag-mask or anaesthetic breathing system.

Further reading
1 Marx, J., Hockberger, R. & Walls, R. (2002) *Rosen's Emergency Medicine – Concepts and Clinical Practice*, 5th edn. St Louis: Mosby.
2 Healy, T. & Knight, P.R. (2003) *Wylie & Churchill-Davidson's A Practice of Anesthesia*, 7th edn. London: Arnold.
3 Walls, R.M., Luten, R.C., Murphy, M.F. & Schneider, R.E. (2004) *Manual of Emergency Airway Management*, 2nd edn. Philadelphia: Lippincott, Williams & Wilkins.
4 Krantz, B., Ali, J., Aprahamian, C. *et al.* (2004) *Advanced Trauma Life Support Course Provider Manual*, 7th edn. Chicago: American College of Surgeons.
5 Nolan, J., Soar, J., Lockey, A. *et al.* (2006) *Advanced Life Support*, 5th edn. London: Resuscitation Council.
6 Roberts, K., Whalley, H. & Bleetman, A. (2005) The nasopharyngeal airway: dispelling myths and establishing the facts. *Emerg Med J*; **22**: 394–6.

5

Indications for intubation

Tim Parke, Dermot McKeown and Colin Graham

Objectives

The objectives of this chapter are to:
- understand that all airway care starts with basic manoeuvres and oxygen
- recognize four situations in which intubation is likely to be required
- be able to distinguish between an immediate need for intubation and an urgent need for intubation
- be aware of important reversible causes of an impaired airway or ventilation.

Introduction

Control of the airway is control of the clinical scenario. Early effective airway care can establish a safe position from which all other priorities flow; conversely, misjudged airway decisions can make a bad situation worse. It is therefore crucial that the practitioner managing the airway formulates a clear plan, communicates this to the team, and calls for help when appropriate.

The decision to intubate or not is often the key first decision in treating a critically ill or injured patient. Tracheal intubation with a cuffed tube secures the airway and enables oxygenation and ventilation of the lungs. It protects the lungs from aspiration of blood or vomit and enables sedation to be safely given without risk of respiratory compromise.

However, the procedure can be technically difficult and failed intubation or a misplaced tracheal tube can be rapidly lethal. The injection of drugs to achieve intubation also carries a further set of pharmacological complications, and commits the patient to ventilatory support.

> Intubation is indicated when the risks of continuing with basic airway support are greater than the risks of intubation

Basic airway manoeuvres always form the mainstay of the immediate management of the emergency airway, however briefly applied.

General considerations

There are four clinical situations in which intubation may be indicated:
1 apnoeic patient in respiratory arrest
2 patient with obstructed/partially obstructed airway where basic airway care is ineffective

Emergency Airway Management, eds. Jonathan Benger, Jerry Nolan and Mike Clancy.
Published by Cambridge University Press. © College of Emergency Medicine, London 2009.

3 patient requiring invasive respiratory support for oxygenation or ventilatory failure

4 patient in whom basic airway care is effective, but whose predicted clinical course includes a high probability of airway obstruction, aspiration or ventilatory failure.

Within these groups there is often considerable overlap, and several indications may coexist. The urgency of the intubation must be decided for each patient. Broadly, there are:

- **immediate intubations**, in which the patient is deteriorating rapidly and definitive airway care is required with a minimum of delay
- **urgent intubations**, in which basic techniques can maintain the physiology of the patient for a short period, pending intubation
- **observant situations**, in which no indication for intubation currently exists, and the patient can be closely observed for any deterioration.

> The initial step of providing supplemental oxygen and basic airway care must never be overlooked

The success of supplemental oxygen and basic airway manoeuvres is critical in deciding both the need for and the urgency of the intubation. For example, a patient in coma with obstruction of an anatomically normal airway can usually be oxygenated for a short period using basic techniques with or without bag-mask support. Urgent intubation may then follow rapidly to prevent respiratory failure and aspiration. Conversely, a patient in coma with facial injuries or vomit in the airway that cannot be adequately oxygenated using basic techniques requires immediate intubation to avoid severe hypoxaemia.

It is also important to carry out an early rapid assessment of the likely technical difficulty of intubation (see Chapter 3). If there is a high risk of failed intubation, then this must be balanced against the assessed urgency of the situation. For example, a patient with partial airway obstruction from a laryngeal malignancy who is well oxygenated is likely to be technically difficult to intubate and can wait for expert assessment and specialist techniques. Conversely, a patient with partial airway obstruction from burns who is hypoxic is also likely to be technically difficult to intubate but requires immediate placement of a definitive airway by the first practitioner with the appropriate skills.

Airway decision-making must not be dissociated from the clinical scenario. In some cases, there may be reversible causes for airway obstruction, respiratory compromise or reduced conscious level. If these are identified, they should be treated while continuing basic airway care. Clearly, if such measures are not rapidly effective, it may be necessary to proceed to definitive airway care. Reversible causes are specified in each of the following sections.

Intubation may not always be appropriate for patients with end-stage diseases. If in doubt, treat, but where time permits obtain further information.

Box 5.1 Reversible causes of airway obstruction or respiratory compromise

---

- arrhythmia (e.g. ventricular fibrillation)
- fitting
- rapidly reversible causes of coma, including hypoglycaemia and opioid overdose
- bronchospasm
- pneumothorax
- left ventricular failure
- anaphylaxis.

Clinical indications for intubation
Apnoeic patient in respiratory arrest

These patients are deeply unconscious with no significant respiratory effort, and often in full cardiorespiratory arrest. Basic airway manoeuvres are instituted and bag-mask ventilation commenced with supplemental high-flow oxygen. Advanced life support protocols are followed.

At a suitable point in the initial resuscitation cycles the patient should be intubated. This enables more effective ventilation and oxygenation, frees up team members from holding the facemask, and prevents further aspiration secondary to distension of the stomach from bag-mask ventilation.

As the patient is profoundly unconscious, attempts at intubation can be carried out without the assistance of induction or paralyzing drugs. The airway reflexes are absent, there is no autonomic response to airway manipulation and the cords are open.

Reversible cause: ventricular fibrillation Attempts at restoring a spontaneous circulation take priority over intubation (but not basic airway care). If output is quickly restored by defibrillation, with a rapid return to consciousness, intubation is not usually required.

Patient with obstructed or partially obstructed airway who does not respond to basic airway manoeuvres

There are groups of patients for whom basic airway techniques are relatively ineffective, and they may require immediate definitive airway placement. These patients are uncommon – not because airway obstruction is uncommon, but because almost all patients can be improved by the judicious application of high-quality basic airway care.

Patients may fall into the immediate category because of:
- anatomical disruption of their airway
- active aspiration of blood or vomit.

These situations are often complicated by reduced conscious level because of hypoxaemia from the obstructed airway, or other coexisting mechanisms (e.g. head injury, overdose). The particular problem with this group is that not only are these patients in need of prompt intubation to prevent hypoxic brain injury, but they can also be technically demanding to intubate. The recognition of such a patient, or prior warning of the arrival of such a patient, should prompt an early call for senior assistance.

Likely clinical scenarios include:

Facial trauma Disruption to normal facial anatomy may render an airway unmaintainable without intubation. This is particularly true of complex midface fractures, where the upper airway is compromised by the displaced bony segment, and of complex jaw fractures, where the tongue loses its normal support and falls back to obstruct the airway.

It may also be impossible to maintain the airway in facial trauma because of severe haemorrhage from facial bones and soft tissues. The patient may be inhaling blood or exsanguinating from blood loss. Packing to stop the bleeding may further compromise the airway.

Patients with complex facial injuries are also often head-injured, rendering them combative or comatose with impaired protective airway reflexes.

The finding of a hypoxic, obtunded trauma patient with severe facial injuries and a compromised airway necessitates an early decision to intubate

While preparations are made, basic airway care and supplemental oxygen are provided. These situations are technically challenging and have a very high potential for failed intubation. Call for senior assistance immediately. Preparations are made for a failed intubation – or rapid conversion to a surgical airway ('plan B').

Laryngeal disruption/swelling Direct injury to the larynx may make the airway impossible to maintain. Blunt trauma to the front of the neck may fracture the larynx and produce stridor, crepitus and surgical emphysema.

Similarly, a penetrating injury to the neck may produce an expanding haematoma that compresses and distorts the airway, causing stridor, hoarseness and respiratory distress.

Infection, anaphylaxis, radiotherapy or burns may cause internal swelling of the larynx or epiglottis. As with external damage to the larynx, this may produce hoarseness, stridor and respiratory distress.

In all these scentarios, the airway is compromised and likely to deteriorate quickly to full obstruction. Stridor in an adult is a particularly worrying sign. Simple airway manoeuvres will not be effective, although supplemental oxygen can buy some time before hypoxaemia occurs.

This situation is extremely hazardous, as the distortion of normal anatomy can make intubation extremely difficult, or impossible. Furthermore, a rescue surgical airway via cricothyroidotomy may also be technically difficult. Summon senior anaesthetic assistance immediately, along with a surgeon capable of performing emergency tracheostomy.

Despite the risks, once the patient begins to become hypoxaemic, intubation must be attempted urgently by the most experienced person present before the patient becomes impossible to intubate. If adequate oxygenation can be achieved using supplemental oxygen, sitting posture and suction, it is safer to defer airway intervention until senior anaesthetic assistance arrives. The balance of risk in these difficult cases depends on the experience and airway skills of the most senior doctor present.

Coma with difficult airway or profuse vomiting Patients may have reduced conscious level through head injury, cerebral haemorrhage, metabolic coma or drug overdose. The airway can usually be maintained for a short period using simple airway techniques, while preparations for intubation are made. The provision of a definitive airway is therefore urgent, rather than immediate.

In some circumstances, however, this is not possible and the airway is unmaintainable, even if anatomically normal. It is important to distinguish these patients as they may require immediate intubation to prevent severe hypoxaemia.

Conditions causing difficulty in maintaining airway in coma may include:
- prolonged seizures
- pre-existing characteristics (limited neck movement, facial hair, obesity)
- active aspiration (vomit or blood in the upper airway).

All these patients may also be difficult to intubate, and this should be taken into account when deciding on the timing of airway management.

The common clinical feature to all of these scenarios is a patient who has an airway that is compromised by fluid (blood, vomit) and/or anatomical disruption. This will manifest as noisy breathing, usually with snoring, gurgling or stridor, and will be associated with marked respiratory distress unless or until the conscious level falls. Later, hypoventilation occurs with reduced air entry progressing to apnoea with weak, tugging respiratory efforts. Hypoxaemia can be a relatively late sign, especially if the patient is receiving supplemental oxygen, and the saturation monitor cannot detect retention of CO_2.

The management of all such patients consists of basic airway care, suction and high-flow oxygen. The response to these initial actions will determine the urgency of proceeding to intubation, coupled with an assessment of the likely technical difficulty in carrying out the procedure.

Reversible causes: fitting, coma, anaphylaxis Even in some very difficult to maintain airways, there may be reversible causes that should be sought, since their presence changes the clinical scenario and in some cases may even avoid the need for intubation. Treat convulsions with intravenous benzodiazepines. Coma caused by hypotension, hypoglycaemia or opioid overdose should be treated urgently. Laryngeal oedema from anaphylaxis may respond to parenteral adrenaline, and laryngeal obstruction caused by haemorrhage within the neck can be relieved in some cases, e.g. after thyroid surgery by opening the surgical wound.

Patient requiring invasive respiratory support for ventilatory failure or critical oxygenation

Patients may require a definitive airway to enable invasive ventilation for respiratory failure. There are two overlapping physiological types of respiratory failure.

Type 1 respiratory failure Failure of oxygenation with no CO_2 retention caused by conditions such as:
- severe chest trauma
- pneumonia
- acute respiratory distress syndrome
- acute pulmonary oedema.

In these cases, there is usually severe V/Q mismatching. A decision to proceed to ventilation is usually taken after attempts at oxygenation by non-invasive means have failed. The respiratory effort made by the patient will often determine the urgency with which respiratory support is instituted. It is preferable to intubate the patient before exhaustion or type 2 respiratory failure supervenes.

Type 2 respiratory failure Failure of ventilation with CO_2 retention caused by conditions such as:
- chronic obstructive pulmonary disease/asthma
- coma/overdose
- neuromuscular disorders.

In these cases hypoventilation with slow or inadequate respiration predominates; oxygenation may be adequate. In mild cases in conscious patients, non-invasive ventilation may be appropriate, but if the conscious level is impaired or the patient becomes severely acidaemic, invasive ventilation is required. In severe cases, the patient may require bag-mask ventilation to maintain adequate gas exchange pending institution of formal respiratory support.

It is not possible to deliver more than 80% oxygen via a facemask, and ventilation of obtunded patients by non-invasive means (including bag-mask) carries a high aspiration risk because of distension of the stomach.

In all these patients, there is usually some time to optimize conditions and fully prepare before intubation. The intubation of patients who are hypoxic and/or acidaemic carries a significant risk of complications.

Reversible causes: bronchospasm, pneumothorax, LVF, opioids Seek potentially reversible causes of respiratory failure and treat while basic support is carried out. Specifically, treat bronchospasm with bronchodilators, pneumothorax with chest drainage, pulmonary oedema with diuretics and nitrates (not opioids in respiratory failure) and where possible, reverse respiratory depressants (e.g. opioids, neuromuscular blocking drugs).

Patients in whom basic airway care is effective, but the predicted clinical course includes high probability of airway obstruction, aspiration or ventilatory failure

Many critically ill patients require intubation because there is a significant risk of adverse events developing. The urgency with which this is required will depend on the predicted clinical course for that patient.

The patients to whom this applies are those with a significant risk of:

- respiratory arrest
- airway obstruction
- aspiration
- respiratory failure.

The patient environment also needs to be considered. There is a greater risk for patients in circumstances where airway interventions cannot be achieved easily, e.g. during transport or CT scanning.

> If the patient has an airway that could become compromised, intubate before transport or scanning

This group includes those patients who require basic airway manoeuvres (e.g. an oropharyngeal airway) to maintain a satisfactory airway. Commonly, they are unconscious patients who have impaired airway protective reflexes with a high risk of aspiration and respiratory depression. It also includes patients who need sedating, in whom there is a high risk of respiratory failure.

Likely clinical scenarios include the following.

Potentially compromised airway anatomy: burns, laryngeal tumour, epiglottitis, anaphylaxis Patients with distortion of their airway caused by malignancy, trauma or infection may present with signs of established airway obstruction; however, they may also present earlier with signs of an airway at risk.

Common examples include:

- neck swelling with penetrating trauma
- hoarseness with facial burns
- tongue swelling with anaphylaxis.

Often, their arterial blood is well oxygenated and they can cope as long as they are sat up and breathe supplemental oxygen. The clinical context must be taken into account. If the airway is likely to deteriorate rapidly, e.g. because of burns or an expanding haematoma, intubate the patient's trachea as soon as possible. If the patient is likely to improve rapidly with treatment, such as in anaphylaxis, then intubation may be replaced with careful observation and immediate effective treatment.

If a patient develops complete airway obstruction and worsening hypoxaemia, intubate immediately using standard RSI techniques.

Head injury/coma Conditions causing reduced consciousness with a particular risk of airway or ventilatory compromise:
- head injury
- intracranial haemorrhage
- overdose (particularly tricyclic antidepressants)
- prolonged seizures
- hepatic encephalopathy.

In the presence of head injury or raised intracranial pressure (ICP), hypoventilation causes hypercapnia and increases cerebral oedema. In these patients airway and ventilatory complications frequently occur during transport to other hospitals, to other clinical areas or in the CT scanner.

> Patients with a Glasgow Coma Scale (GCS) of 8 or less are at very high risk of aspiration because of loss of airway reflexes. They also frequently have abnormalities of respiratory drive with a tendency to hypoventilation and respiratory arrest

Treatment of these patients starts with basic airway manoeuvres and supplemental oxygen. If the airway cannot be maintained immediate intubation is required. Otherwise, if it is clear that there are no immediately reversible causes for the coma, make preparations for intubation. Ensure the patient is pre-oxygenated adequately and positioned optimally. Hypotension is also potentially harmful, particularly in head injury: ensure cardiovascular stability before intubation (see Trauma and raised intracranial pressure in Chapter 11 for further information).

Impaired consciousness with agitation Patients with a GCS of 9–12 may need to be intubated, even if there is no airway obstruction and no ventilatory failure. Obtunded, agitated patients, particularly those who have suffered multiple injuries, including head injuries, can be exceptionally difficult to manage without anaesthesia. This is because procedures such as CT scanning become impossible, and placing lines and tubes hazardous; furthermore, many of these patients will deteriorate and are at risk of developing airway obstruction, hypoventilation and aspiration.

In this group, it is essential to first seek reversible causes of agitation, such as pain, shock, hypoglycaemia or a full bladder. If none are present and the predicted clinical course is that the patient is likely to remain unmanageable, then RSI and intubation should be considered. This is particularly the case for highly agitated head-injured patients, who are at risk of becoming comatose with very little warning.

Intubating an unco-operative patient also carries considerable risks. Inadequate pre-oxygenation, loss of venous access and sub-optimal positioning are all potential factors that may contribute to intubation difficulty. In some cases, sedation may be required to control the situation before undertaking a formal RSI.

Severe shock with acidosis Some critically ill patients with septic shock can develop intractable acidosis and impaired consciousness, which necessitates ventilatory support. Attempts at improving the shock state with supplemental oxygen, fluid resuscitation and inotropes form the mainstay of initial management. However, if it is clear that the patient's clinical course is deteriorating, consider intubation to optimize oxygenation, remove the work of breathing and assist in the correction of metabolic acidosis.

Careful calculation of the dose of induction drug is essential because severe hypotension is common. If possible, intubate these patients with invasive arterial monitoring established, and with the involvement of experienced intensivist staff.

The common feature of all of these patients is that on initial assessment they either do not require, or improve significantly with, basic airway manoeuvres and supplemental oxygen. Although this implies that the need for intubation is not immediate, they may still be candidates for emergency intubation. Patients may deteriorate quickly: e.g. a burns patient may develop stridor and hypoxaemia, a head-injured patient may fit or vomit, and a septic patient may develop severe respiratory distress. These events upgrade the clinical situation to an immediate need for intubation. However, as many of these scenarios are accompanied by considerable intubation risks, some investment of time in organizing experienced personnel and suitable equipment, together with adequate preparation of the patient, is both possible and desirable.

Reversible causes: hypoglycaemia and fitting Some patients with impaired conscious level are likely to have a benign clinical course, such as those who are hypoglycaemic or post-ictal. These patients do not require intubation unless they do not respond rapidly to treatment.

Summary
- Intubation is indicated when:
  a the risks of continuing basic airway support exceed the risks of intubation
  b there are no rapidly reversible factors.
- Intubation is always preceded by basic airway care and supplemental oxygen.
- Immediate intubation is required if basic techniques cannot provide adequate oxygenation.

Further reading
1 Resuscitation Council: Advanced life support guidelines
   www.resus.org.uk/pages/als.htm
2 Trauma.Org: Airway management of the trauma victim
   www.trauma.org/anaesthesia/airway.html

3 British Thoracic Society: Non-invasive ventilation guidelines
   www.brit-thoracic.org.uk/docs/NIV.pdf
4 Intensive Care Society: Guidelines for the transport of the critically ill adult
   www.ics.ac.uk/downloads/icstransport2002mem.pdf
5 Neuro-Anaesthesia Society: Recommendations for the transfer of patients
   with acute head injuries to neurosurgical units
   www.nasgbi.org.uk/docs/headinj5.htm

Preparation for rapid sequence induction and tracheal intubation

Nikki Maran, Neil Nichol and Simon Leigh-Smith

Objectives

The objectives of this chapter are to understand how to:

- prepare thoroughly for rapid sequence induction (RSI) and tracheal intubation
- position patients optimally to maximize the success of laryngoscopy and intubation
- assemble and check the equipment and drugs required for RSI and tracheal intubation
- use appropriate monitoring and know its strengths and limitations
- reassess the patient rapidly and ascertain all the required information before undertaking RSI
- identify and use team resources appropriately to maximize team co-operation and understanding.

Introduction

Making the decision that a patient requires a rapid sequence induction (RSI) is the entry point to the sequence of preparation for this procedure. While there may be times when intubation of the patient needs to be achieved immediately, there are very few instances in which placement of the tracheal tube is so time critical that these basic preparatory steps cannot be followed. With a systematic approach and good team working, this will take only a few minutes and avoid many possible problems and complications.

The PEACH approach (Box 6.1) provides a useful mnemonic.

Positioning

Correct positioning of the patient's head and neck improves the view of the larynx at laryngoscopy and the likelihood of successful intubation. Alignment of the oral, pharyngeal and laryngeal axes during laryngoscopy provides a clear view from the incisors to the laryngeal inlet (see Chapter 4).

Approximately 20% of RSI undertaken in the emergency department require stabilization of the cervical spine: in almost all other cases the patient should be placed in the optimum intubating position, unless spinal deformity or arthritis makes this impractical or inadvisable.

Emergency Airway Management, eds. Jonathan Benger, Jerry Nolan and Mike Clancy.
Published by Cambridge University Press. © College of Emergency Medicine, London 2009.

Box 6.1 The PEACH mnemonic

Positioning
Equipment – including drugs
Attach – oxygen and monitoring
Checks – resuscitation, brief history, intravenous access and neurology
Help – who is available and what are the abilities of the team?

Equipment

Prepare and check thoroughly all equipment before undertaking any anaesthetic: these checks are the responsibility of the practitioner who will give the anaesthetic. This individual must be familiar with all the equipment and check it adequately. Many of these checks may be undertaken in advance as part of a routine daily check. A systematic approach is recommended (Box 6.2): equipment is placed in a logical sequence and positioned conveniently within easy reach. An example of this is shown in Figure 6.1. Equipment for managing a failed intubation must also be readily available and checked.

Trolley

Check the patient trolley/stretcher to ensure operation of the height adjustment and mechanism for rapid tilting. Position it optimally to ensure access to the patient for intubation, effortless view of monitoring and immediate availability of the anaesthetic equipment.

Suction

Suction should generate a negative pressure of 400 cmH$_2$O within ten seconds when obstructed. It should be immediately accessible during management of the airway, and is usually placed under the pillow on the right-hand side.

Rigid catheters are required for suctioning of the upper airway (e.g. Yankauer type), and flexible suction catheters for suctioning down the tracheal tube after placement.

Oxygen delivery apparatus

Check oxygen delivery systems for patency and ability to generate positive pressure for ventilation. Check also the function of adjustable pressure limiting (APL) valves.

Connect a heat and moisture exchanger (HME) filter to the breathing system: it prevents contamination of ventilation equipment and helps to warm and humidify the oxygen-enriched air in the trachea. Check that all connections are hand tight.

Airway adjuncts

Airway adjuncts, including several sizes of oral and nasopharyngeal airways, should be available. Take care when removing these devices from wrappers: avoid sealing the ends of the airways with a thin film of polythene.

Box 6.2 Equipment for rapid sequence induction and tracheal intubation

Basic resuscitation equipment
- Tilting trolley/stretcher
- Oxygen delivery apparatus including mask with reservoir and oxygen tubing
- Suction:
  - wide-bore suction tubing
  - rigid suction catheter
  - flexible suction catheter – sized appropriately for other airway equipment
- Airway adjuncts:
  - nasopharyngeal airway (sizes 6 and 7)
  - oropharyngeal airway (sizes 2, 3 and 4)
- Intravenous access equipment
- Monitors

Advanced airway equipment
- Pre-oxygenation/ventilation breathing system:
  - Mapleson C or equivalent anaesthetic breathing system
  - bag-mask apparatus with reservoir bag and oxygen tubing
  - filter (heat and moisture exchanger)
- Drugs – in labelled syringes
- Laryngoscope handles and blades (sizes 3 and 4 for adults)
- Magill's forceps
- Intubating stylet, bougie and KY jelly
- Tracheal tubes in a range of sizes
- 20 ml syringe
- Tie and adhesive tape
- Equipment for patient ventilation:
  - catheter mount
  - colourimetric end-tidal CO_2 detector
  - quantitative end-tidal CO_2 monitor
- Ventilator

Failed intubation equipment
- Laryngeal mask airway (LMA) (sizes 3, 4 and 5)
  - 50 ml syringe connected to LMA
  - water-soluble jelly
- Surgical cricothyroidotomy set
- Needle cricothyroidotomy kit with high-pressure injector

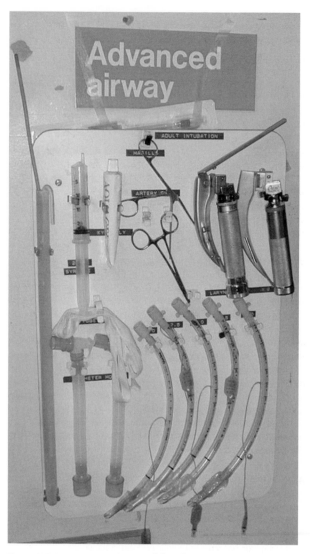

Figure 6.1 An emergency airway grab board.

Laryngoscopes

The curved Macintosh laryngoscope blade is commonly available in sizes 3 (short) and 4 (long); use the size 4 blade in all but the smallest adult patients. Check that the laryngoscope light is adequately bright before starting an RSI. Alternative laryngoscope blades such as the McCoy blade (which enables further elevation of the epiglottis using the lever on the tip of the curved blade) or the Miller straight-bladed laryngoscope are useful alternatives. Use of these alternative blades requires adequate training: they should never be used for the first time in a difficult situation.

Tracheal tubes

The tracheal tube sizes recommended for adults are 7.0 or 7.5 mm for women and 8.0 mm for men; however, a range of tracheal tube sizes should be available. While tubes are normally cut to length (22–24 cm for women, 24–26 cm for men), if facial swelling is likely, e.g. with burns, blunt facial trauma or anaphylaxis, leave the tube uncut. A syringe must be available to fill the cuff with air, and this should be checked to ensure that it does not leak.

Bougies and stylets

The bougie and stylet are very useful aids to intubation. If the view at laryngoscopy is less than perfect (grade 3 or a difficult grade 2), an intubating bougie can be inserted behind the epiglottis and into the trachea, and a tracheal tube then railroaded into position over the bougie. Some practitioners prefer to use an intubating stylet: the rigidity of this device enables the tube to be shaped to bring the tip more anterior, forming a 'J' shape to facilitate intubation. For further information see Chapter 7.

Ventilation system

Carefully check the ventilation system and all its connections according to the manufacturer's instructions. Check the system functions normally and check the settings of the high and low pressure alarms, the ventilation mode, respiratory rate, tidal volume, inspiratory:expiratory (I:E) ratio and positive end expiratory pressure (PEEP) (see Chapter 10 for further information).

Equipment for failed intubation

Check the equipment for failed intubation and place it in an easily accessible location during all intubations.

Drugs

The choice of drugs for induction of anaesthesia and maintenance of sedation and analgesia are described in detail in Chapter 8. Once the drugs are selected, prepare them in appropriately sized, clearly labelled syringes. Include the drugs that may be required for treatment of any hypotension associated with the RSI.

Attach
Oxygen
Give high concentration oxygen to the patient in all but the most unusual circumstances: use a breathing system that will maximize oxygen delivery. In the case of pre-oxygenation, this may entail using an anaesthetic breathing system. An alternative would be a bag-mask with a functioning oxygen reservoir.

Monitoring
The Association of Anaesthetists of Great Britain and Ireland has defined minimum recommended standards of monitoring, which are required wherever anaesthesia is administered (see Further reading section). These standards apply as much outside the operating theatre as they do within it, and include the monitoring of:
- inspired oxygen concentration (FiO_2)
- capnometry
- pulse oximetry
- non-invasive blood pressure
- continuous electrocardiograph (ECG).

Anyone carrying out anaesthesia should understand the rationale behind these recommendations and the major strengths and limitations of the different monitors that they are likely to use on a regular basis.

Oxygen analyzer
Use an oxygen analyzer to ensure adequate delivery of oxygen whenever positive pressure ventilation is undertaken. Measurement of FiO_2 is often achieved in combination with measurement of end tidal CO_2.

Electrocardiograph
ECG monitoring is an easy and non-invasive method for detecting changes in heart rate and rhythm. Changes in morphology of the ECG may indicate myocardial ischaemia or electrolyte disturbances such as hypo- or hyperkalaemia. The ECG gives no indication of cardiac output.

Non-invasive blood pressure
Measurement of the blood pressure alone provides limited information about tissue perfusion; however, trends may indicate physiological change and sudden hypotension may warn of an acute life-threatening event such as anaphylaxis, tension pneumothorax, etc. Blood pressure is measured non-invasively by an inflatable cuff of the correct size on the upper arm. Measurement should be more frequent when physiological change is anticipated, such as at the induction of anaesthesia. These machines are notoriously unreliable at the extremes of pressure and with irregular rhythms. In these circumstances, direct measurement of blood pressure using an intra-arterial cannula is preferable.

Pulse oximetry

The nature of the plethysmograph trace gives information about the state of the peripheral circulation. Pulsatile flow is required for correct function: in low flow states the information displayed by the pulse oximeter may be inaccurate. While the pulse oximeter indicates oxygenation, it may not reflect adequacy of ventilation of the patient: information should be interpreted in conjunction with capnography and arterial blood gas analysis.

Capnography

Measurement of expired CO_2 is the most reliable way of ensuring that the tracheal tube is in the airway, and must be used during every anaesthetic. Trends in CO_2 will indicate the adequacy of ventilation. A sudden fall in CO_2 may indicate misplacement of the tracheal tube or a reduced cardiac output.

Checks
Resuscitation

As treatment progresses, review airway, breathing and circulation (ABC), paying particular attention to any potentially reversible problems. Request any relevant laboratory tests and optimize the drug treatment of any medical conditions, including analgesia if appropriate. Document all baseline physiology.

Brief history

Review a brief history (such as the AMPLE history described in Box 6.3) to obtain information relevant to clinical decisions.

Box 6.3 AMPLE history

- **A**llergies
- **M**edications
- **P**MHx (past medical history)
- **L**ast
  - anaesthetic (complications)
  - meal
  - tetanus
- **E**vents
  - leading up to this situation

Intravenous access

Ensure that there are two large-bore functioning intravenous (IV) lines before giving any anaesthetic drugs. Failure of the sole IV line during an RSI is dangerous.

Neurology

Undertake a brief neurological examination before induction of anaesthesia (and therefore abolition of neurological signs). This will include assessment of GCS, pupil signs and presence of abnormal posturing. Look for diaphragmatic breathing, inappropriate vasodilatation or priapism. Document all neurological findings.

Help
Call for help

An appropriately experienced individual should be present before undertaking advanced airway care in a critically ill patient. If advanced airway care is anticipated, summon expert help immediately. The presence of a senior emergency airway practitioner from the earliest opportunity is ideal.

Rapid sequence induction of anaesthesia outside the operating theatre requires a minimum of three or four staff. One practitioner takes responsibility for the airway and another oversees the clinical care of the patient. The airway practitioner will require an assistant who is capable of applying cricoid pressure correctly, and who has knowledge of the equipment and techniques to be used, including the plan for difficult or failed intubation. A fourth member of staff will be required to undertake manual in-line stabilization of the cervical spine, if this is indicated.

Team dynamics and leadership

Teams normally comprise individuals who are familiar with working together. While this may be true of the staff within a single hospital department, the presence of numerous staff from different disciplines, often with differing attitudes, creates a more complex dynamic. In this situation, good team leadership is vitally important. The key skills of good leadership include:
- good briefing of new team members
- delegation
- allocation and agreement of roles
- task distribution (and support if required)
- co-ordination and communication.

Review and feedback

A debrief of team performance after the event provides an opportunity for reflection and learning.

Summary

Thorough preparation before undertaking RSI and tracheal intubation will minimize unexpected problems and facilitate a smooth and successful procedure.

Further reading

1 Association of Anaesthetists of Great Britain and Ireland (2000) *Recommendations for Standards of Monitoring*, 3rd edn. London: Association of Anaesthetists of Great Britain and Ireland. www.aagbi.org/guidelines.html

Rapid sequence induction and tracheal intubation

Neil Nichol, Nikki Maran and Simon Leigh-Smith

Objectives

The objectives of this chapter are to understand:

- the importance of pre-oxygenation
- the technique of rapid sequence induction (RSI) of anaesthesia and tracheal intubation
- the confirmation of successful intubation
- the importance of immediate review of patient physiology after intubation.

Introduction

Rapid sequence induction of anaesthesia (RSI) involves injecting an anaesthetic induction drug to achieve hypnosis, rapidly followed by a neuromuscular blocking drug to produce complete paralysis. To prevent inflation of the stomach, the lungs are not usually ventilated between induction and intubation, and the airway is protected by applying cricoid pressure to prevent regurgitation of gastric contents. The time from loss of consciousness to securing the airway is minimized because the patient's stomach is assumed to be full.

Pre-oxygenation

Effective pre-oxygenation replaces the nitrogen in the alveoli with oxygen, which increases the oxygen reserve in the lung. Pre-oxygenation maximizes the time before desaturation occurs following the onset of apnoea. This provides more time for intubation to be attempted before having to stop to re-oxygenate the patient's lungs (see Chapter 2). Whenever possible, give 100% oxygen for three minutes before induction of anaesthesia. A patient who is breathing inadequately may not achieve enough alveolar ventilation to replace nitrogen in the lungs with oxygen. These patients may therefore require assisted ventilation to achieve adequate pre-oxygenation before RSI.

The time to desaturation is related not only to the effectiveness of the pre-oxygenation phase, but also to the age and weight of the patient and their physiological status. In a healthy adult the time taken for arterial blood to desaturate to 90% may be as long as eight minutes after effective pre-oxygenation. This time is significantly reduced in critically ill patients, partly because full pre-oxygenation often cannot be achieved (see Figure 2.11).

Emergency Airway Management, eds. Jonathan Benger, Jerry Nolan and Mike Clancy. Published by Cambridge University Press. © College of Emergency Medicine, London 2009.

The shape of the oxyhaemoglobin dissociation curve (Figure 2.12) indicates that the rate of decline of oxygen saturation is greatest below 92%; once the pulse oximeter indicates a SpO_2 of 92% or less, the patient's lungs should be ventilated immediately with 100% oxygen.

It is not normal practice to assist ventilation during RSI until tracheal intubation has been accomplished, but if the patient requires assisted ventilation before induction it is reasonable to continue this after the induction drug has been given and while awaiting the onset of neuromuscular blockade. This is particularly true for patients who desaturate rapidly when assisted ventilation is discontinued.

Careful preparation and full pre-oxygenation buy time during RSI

The technique of rapid sequence induction

Adequate preparation will have been completed (acronym PEACH: see Chapter 6) and the patient pre-oxygenated. The induction drug produces unconsciousness, and is followed immediately by a neuromuscular blocking drug, using a pre-calculated dose. Both drugs are injected rapidly into a functioning intravenous line with an infusion running to expedite drug delivery. If an assistant gives the drugs, good communication is required to ensure that the dose and timing of injection are thoroughly understood.

Cricoid pressure

A trained assistant applies cricoid pressure as the induction drug is injected and consciousness lost. The cricoid ring is identified (below the thyroid cartilage and cricothyroid membrane) and stabilized between the thumb and middle finger. Firm pressure is then applied to the centre of the cricoid cartilage using the index finger, pressing directly backwards to compress the upper oesophagus between the cricoid and the cervical vertebra posteriorly (Figure 7.1). Applied correctly, this will prevent passive reflux of gastric contents into the pharynx. The correct pressure is 30–40 Newtons, which is enough to be painful in a conscious patient. Inadequate pressure will not occlude the oesophagus; however, excessive force or incorrect placement will deform the larynx and make laryngoscopy and intubation more difficult (see Chapter 9). Cricoid pressure should not be applied in the presence of active vomiting, because it may cause oesophageal rupture. There is no evidence that a second hand applied behind the neck (two-handed cricoid pressure) in an attempt to restrict cervical spine movement is any safer than the standard technique. Cricoid pressure is removed only on the instruction of the intubating clinician once correct tube placement has been confirmed.

Laryngoscopy and intubation

The laryngoscope is held in the left hand, and the tip of the blade inserted into the right side of the patient's mouth. It may be necessary to adjust the hand of

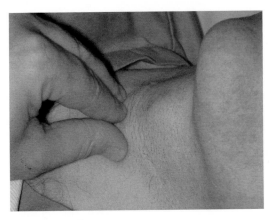

Figure 7.1 Cricoid pressure.

the assistant applying cricoid pressure to enable the handle of the laryngoscope to be placed correctly as the blade is inserted into the mouth. The blade is advanced further into the oropharynx, and gradually toward the midline, keeping the tongue anteriorly and displacing it to the left. When the epiglottis is seen, the blade tip is placed superiorly in the vallecula, and the epiglottis lifted by elevation of the laryngoscope in the line of the handle (see Figure 7.2). The laryngeal inlet is seen anterior to the arytenoid cartilages, and the vocal cords identified. Suction may be required to improve the view. Identifying the tip of the epiglottis is key to this process, and should be sought specifically at each intubation attempt. 'Levering' the handle of the laryngoscope backwards will damage the teeth or soft tissues of the mouth, and will not improve the view.

The laryngeal view is classified according to the Cormack and Lehane grading system (Figure 3.1).

Use rigid suction to clear any secretions, blood or vomit before passing the tracheal tube through the cords under direct vision. Use of an intubating stylet or bougie will increase the likelihood of successful intubation, particularly if the patient's head and neck are immobilized.

1 The intubating stylet, preformed into a J shape, is used routinely by some practitioners. The introducer should never protrude beyond the distal end of the tracheal tube, and should be withdrawn after the tip of the tube has passed through the vocal cords; this minimizes the risk of damaging the trachea. The tracheal tube is then advanced until the black line just proximal to the tube cuff lies at or just beyond the vocal cords. Sometimes clockwise rotation of the tube through 45 degrees as it is inserted into the mouth can improve the view: this enables the progress of the tube tip to be followed without the view being obscured by the proximal end of the tube.

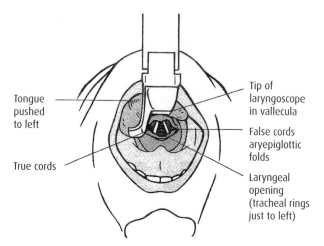

Tongue pushed to left

True cords

Tip of laryngoscope in vallecula

False cords aryepiglottic folds

Laryngeal opening (tracheal rings just to left)

Figure 7.2 The expected view during laryngoscopy.

2 The intubating bougie is invaluable for assisting intubation when the view of the larynx is poor (grade 3 or a difficult grade 2). The tip of the intubating bougie is bent to form an elbow (coudé), shaped like a hockey stick. With the laryngoscope in place, the bougie is passed behind the epiglottis and into the trachea. Detection of clicks as the bougie slides over the tracheal rings helps to confirm correct placement: hold-up of the bougie in the distal airways provides secondary confirmation of placement. While the practitioner maintains the best possible view of the larynx the tracheal tube is then railroaded over the bougie into the trachea: this requires the tracheal tube to be threaded over the bougie by an assistant until they are able to grasp the end protruding from the tracheal tube and hold the bougie still, while the practitioner advances the tracheal tube over the bougie under direction vision. Rotation of the tracheal tube 90 degrees counter-clockwise may ease passage through the cords. While grasping the tracheal tube firmly, the assistant removes the bougie and correct placement is confirmed using the methods described below. Both the practitioner and assistant must be trained and practised in the use of an intubating bougie. Common errors include advancing the tube into the trachea before the assistant has grasped the free end of the bougie, and failure to maintain the best possible laryngeal view while railroading the tracheal tube.

If the laryngeal inlet and vocal cords cannot be seen immediately, the following interventions may improve the grade of view:

• If the blade is too short, select a longer bladed laryngoscope. A shorter laryngoscope blade is required only very rarely; thus, it is sensible to select a size 4 laryngoscope blade from the start.

- Backward, upward and rightward pressure (BURP) on the larynx by an assistant may improve the view. The BURP manoeuvre is different to cricoid pressure, though the two may be applied together.
- Incorrect application of cricoid pressure may obscure the view: if the measures described previously do not enable the larynx to be seen, cautiously relaxing the cricoid pressure with the laryngoscope in place may bring the vocal cords into view.

Once placed correctly in the trachea, the length of the tube at the teeth is noted, and the laryngoscope is removed. The pilot balloon is inflated until no air leak can be heard during inflation of the lungs, and correct placement of the tube is confirmed using the following methods.

Confirmation of tracheal tube placement

Carbon dioxide detection is the gold standard by which placement of the tracheal tube in the airway is confirmed: it must be undertaken routinely, using an end tidal capnometer or, in remote situations, a disposable colourimetric CO_2 detector. The following additional checks are carried out by attaching the breathing system to the tracheal tube and ventilating the patient's lungs manually, but do not by themselves confirm correct tube placement.

- Inspect the chest wall looking for symmetry of movement on ventilation.
- Use a stethoscope to listen in both axillae for air entry.

Once tracheal intubation is confirmed, release the cricoid pressure and secure the tube with a ribbon tie. In a patient with raised intracranial pressure use of adhesive tape instead of a tie will avoid compression of the jugular veins, which has the potential to impair venous drainage and increase intracranial pressure. However, this theoretical risk must be weighed against the possibility of tube displacement as the patient is transported around the hospital or to another hospital. It is good practice to insert an appropriately sized oropharyngeal airway adjacent to the tracheal tube: this reduces the risk of the patient biting on the tube and occluding the airway, and may also be useful if the patient is accidentally extubated.

Capnography must be used wherever RSI occurs

Post-intubation review

The patient is now reassessed, with specific evaluation of the airway, ventilation and circulation. Use a suction catheter to clear material from the lower airways. Check the monitors for heart rate, SpO_2, blood pressure, end tidal CO_2 and peak inspiratory pressure. Request a chest X-ray: it is the responsibility of the intubating clinician to examine the chest film, check the position of the tube and to withdraw or advance the tracheal tube as required.

The stages of rapid sequence induction of anaesthesia and tracheal intubation are summarized in Figure 7.3.

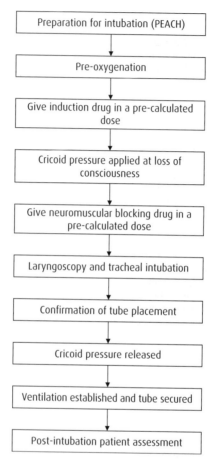

Figure 7.3 The stages of rapid sequence induction of anaesthesia.

Hypotension after rapid sequence induction and intubation

Hypotension occurs commonly after RSI, particularly in the presence of hypovolaemia. There are four common causes.

- Induction drug. This is by far the commonest cause of hypotension immediately following RSI, and is dose related. The induction drug causes hypotension mainly by vasodilatation, but also by myocardial depression. Give fluid 500–1000 ml rapidly and reassess the blood pressure. Give a vasoconstrictor, such as ephedrine or adrenaline, if the hypotension does not respond immediately to fluid. When there is any suspicion of hypovolaemia before induction of anaesthesia give 500–1000 ml fluid rapidly before and during the pre-oxygenation phase: have vasopressor drugs ready to give immediately and, whenever possible, monitor blood pressure continuously using an arterial cannula.

- Hyperventilation with air trapping, often in the context of acute or chronic obstructive airways disease. The peak inspiratory pressure (P_{max}) is high, and the chest may be obviously hyperinflated. It is easy to cause hyperventilation and air trapping in an unwell patient who has desaturated during a difficult intubation. However, the high intra-thoracic pressure impairs venous return to the heart and the cardiac output decreases. A period of disconnection of the breathing system from the tracheal tube will enable adequate time for exhalation of trapped alveolar gas. Continue positive pressure ventilation with a reduced rate and longer expiratory time. Use bronchodilators to relieve bronchospasm. A fluid challenge of 500–1000 ml will help to restore adequate preload.

- Tension pneumothorax. This is uncommon, but potentially catastrophic, and requires rapid recognition and treatment. The earliest signs in a ventilated patient are usually hypoxaemia followed by hypotension. Peak inspiratory pressure may be high, causing difficulty in ventilating the patient's lungs. Clinical signs of a pneumothorax may be detectable: tracheal shift and venous distension in the neck are late and unreliable signs, though they help to confirm the diagnosis if present. Careful examination of the chest before intubation will enable easier detection of the change in air entry after the procedure. Treatment is immediate needle decompression followed by insertion of a chest drain.

- Cardiogenic. Having excluded other causes, the possibility of poor myocardial function should be considered. A 12-lead ECG and urgent echocardiography may be helpful. Monitor the central venous pressure and give fluids and vasoactive drugs as indicated.

Summary

- Successful completion of RSI and tracheal intubation depends on careful preparation and attention to each stage, with effective use of the team as a resource.
- Before embarking on this procedure, the practitioner must be fully prepared for a failed intubation.

Further reading

1 Association of Anaesthetists of Great Britain and Ireland (2000) *Recommendations for Standards of Monitoring*, 3rd edn. London: Association of Anaesthetists of Great Britain and Ireland. See: www.aagbi.org/guidelines.html

2 Walls, R.M. (1993) Rapid-sequence intubation in head trauma. *Ann Emerg Med*; **22**: 1008–13.

3 Reid, C., Chan, L. & Tweeddale, M. (2004) The who, where, and what of RSI: prospective observational study of emergency RSI outside the operating theatre. *Emerg Med J*; **21**: 296–301.

4 Mort, T.C. (2004) Emergency tracheal intubation: complications associated with repeated laryngoscopic attempts. *Anesth Analg*; **99**: 607–13.

8

Pharmacology of emergency airway drugs

Neil Nichol, Nikki Maran and Jonathan Benger

Objectives

The objectives of this chapter are to:

- be familiar with the choice of induction, analgesic and neuromuscular blocking drugs
- understand the advantages and disadvantages of drugs used in emergency airway management
- understand the basic pharmacology of these drugs
- be aware of the possible complications caused by these drugs.

Introduction

The term 'triad of anaesthesia' is used to describe the components of a balanced anaesthetic:

- hypnosis
- analgesia
- muscle relaxation.

The pharmacology of drugs used commonly in emergency airway management will be considered under these three headings.

In unmodified rapid sequence induction (RSI) an analgesic is omitted and the patient is given a pre-calculated dose of induction drug and neuromuscular blocker only. The rationale behind this is that, should intubation fail, the patient will recover from anaesthesia and paralysis quickly, returning to spontaneous ventilation. Opioids, particularly in high doses, will increase the time to spontaneous ventilation. Some patients may have received analgesia before the induction of anaesthesia (e.g. for pain relief in trauma), and under some circumstances it is appropriate to consider modifying an RSI to include a carefully selected dose of opioid given before the induction drug (e.g. RSI in the presence of raised intracranial pressure: see Trauma and raised intracranial pressure in Chapter 11). Opioids are also useful after intubation, when they may be used in combination with a hypnotic to maintain anaesthesia and reduce sympathetic stimulation.

Midazolam is not considered an induction drug in the UK; however, it may occasionally be given by an experienced practitioner to sedate an agitated and unco-operative patient to facilitate the process of RSI. It is also used for procedural sedation, and is therefore included in the hypnosis section.

Emergency Airway Management, eds. Jonathan Benger, Jerry Nolan and Mike Clancy.
Published by Cambridge University Press. © College of Emergency Medicine, London 2009.

Any modification of a standard RSI will alter the pharmacodynamic response to induction drugs. Therefore the risks and benefits of RSI modification should be considered for individual patients.

Hypnosis
Induction drugs

The ideal anaesthetic induction drug would induce anaesthesia smoothly and rapidly without causing pain on injection. It would cause minimal depression of the respiratory and cardiovascular systems, and protect the cerebral circulation. Recovery would be rapid and the drug would have no adverse effects. Unfortunately, such a drug does not exist, and the attributes and limitations of available drugs, as well as the condition of the patient, will determine the final choice. Familiarity with the properties of a specific drug is also very important. It is not appropriate to use an unfamiliar drug for the first time in an emergency.

All induction drugs have the potential to cause hypotension to a greater or lesser extent, particularly when the patient is physiologically compromised.

In the UK, one of four induction drugs are used in emergency RSI: these are summarized in Table 8.1, and described in more detail subsequently. However, this manual does not attempt to provide a comprehensive account of the properties of individual drugs and readers are referred to pharmacological texts for further information.

Etomidate has fewer adverse effects on the cardiovascular system than thiopental or propofol and, particularly in the presence of hypovolaemia, will cause less hypotension than these drugs. In critically ill patients a single dose of etomidate causes adrenal suppression for up to 24 hours: the clinical significance of this is unclear, but it may be a cause of subsequent morbidity in some patient groups. Many practitioners prefer to use thiopental or propofol, even in hypovolaemic patients, but this necessitates considerable experience of these drugs, and a carefully considered dose reduction. Where time allows, the placement of an arterial cannula is invaluable during RSI to provide accurate and continuous blood pressure measurement. Ketamine is a useful induction drug in some circumstances: it is a bronchodilator, causes less hypotension and respiratory depression than the other induction drugs, and is a potent analgesic. It can, however, cause hypertension and is relatively contraindicated in head injury.

Etomidate
Indications
- Induction of anaesthesia in the haemodynamically compromised patient.

Induction characteristics
- 5–15 seconds onset
- 5–15 minutes full recovery
- Myoclonic movement on injection (may be mistaken for seizures)
- Pain on injection.

Table 8.1. Summary of the four commonly used induction drugs

Induction drug	Dose	Onset of anaesthesia	Recovery	Cardiovascular depression	Specific effects
Etomidate	$0.3\,mg\,kg^{-1}$	5–15 seconds	5–15 minutes	+	• Myoclonic movements on induction • Adrenal suppression
Propofol	1.5–$2.5\,mg\,kg^{-1}$	20–40 seconds	5–10 minutes	+++	• Marked hypotension in cardiovascular compromise • Induction agent most commonly used in elective anaesthesia • Pain on injection • Involuntary movements on induction • Anticonvulsant properties
Thiopental	2–$7\,mg\,kg^{-1}$	5–15 seconds	5–15 minutes	++	• Cerebroprotective action • Useful in isolated head injury • Effective anticonvulsant
Ketamine	1–$2\,mg\,kg^{-1}$	15–30 seconds	15–30 minutes	Minimal	• Dissociative state • Potent analgesic • Hypertension • Emergence phenomena e.g. agitation, hallucinations • Bronchodilator • Useful in acute asthma, hypovolaemic trauma and burns

Physiological effects
- Hypnotic
- Relative haemodynamic stability
- Attenuation of the increase in intracranial pressure (ICP) that accompanies laryngoscopy
- Reduced cerebral blood flow
- Reduced cerebral oxygen demand
- Adrenocortical suppression: must never be given by infusion.

Dose
- 0.3 mg kg^{-1} IV.

Propofol
Indications
- Most commonly used induction drug in elective anaesthesia
- Can be used by infusion for maintenance of anaesthesia or sedation
- Sedation in intubated patients on ICU or during transport.

Induction characteristics
- Slow onset (20–40 seconds) can lead to the administration of a drug dose that is relatively too large for the patient
- Rapid return of consciousness.

Physiological effects
- Hypotension is common, and may be severe in cardiovascular compromise; it is caused mainly by vasodilatation but also by a direct myocardial depressant effect
- Apnoea after induction dose
- Pain on injection with some preparations (reduced if 2 ml of 1% lidocaine is mixed with the induction dose or injected before induction)
- Occasional severe bradycardia
- Induction often associated with involuntary movements, but anticonvulsant properties have been demonstrated on electroencephalogram (EEG) studies.

Dose
- 1.5–2.5 mg kg^{-1} IV.

Thiopental sodium
Indications
- Haemodynamically stable patient with:
  - isolated head injury
  - seizures.

Induction characteristics
- 5–15 seconds onset
- 5–15 minutes to recovery.

Physiological effects
- Neuro-inhibition (at barbiturate receptor as part of GABA–receptor complex)
- Cerebroprotective, because of a dose dependent decrease in:
  - cerebral metabolic oxygen consumption
  - cerebral blood flow
  - ICP
- Maintenance of cerebral perfusion pressure
- Venodilatation
- Myocardial depression
- Central respiratory depression.

Dose
- $2-7\,mg\,kg^{-1}$ IV
- Dose reduced to $1.5-2\,mg\,kg^{-1}$ IV in haemodynamically unstable patients.

Ketamine
Indications
- Burns
- Cardiovascularly compromised patient
- Severe bronchospasm.

Induction characteristics
- 15–30 seconds onset when given IV
- Lack of a defined end-point makes dose calculation difficult
- Rapidly absorbed: therefore fast onset when injected IM
- Excitatory phenomena.

Physiological effects
- Profound analgesia
- Sedation
- Dissociative state
- Amnesia (less than benzodiazepines)
- Central sympathetic stimulation leading to:
  - increased heart rate
  - increased blood pressure
- Bronchial smooth muscle relaxation
- Myocardial depression (in doses $>1.5\,mg\,kg^{-1}$)
- Respiratory depression – dose related
- Enhanced laryngeal reflexes, with potential for laryngospasm
- Secretions increased – pharyngeal and bronchial
- Emergence phenomena
  - commoner in adults
  - reduced by pre-treatment with midazolam.

Dose
- 1–$2\,mg\,kg^{-1}$ IV
- $5\,mg\,kg^{-1}$ IM.

Midazolam

Midazolam is a water-soluble benzodiazepine that has anxiolytic, sedative and anticonvulsant properties. At physiological pH midazolam is lipid soluble and reaches the central nervous system quickly. It has a shorter duration of action than most other benzodiazepines, but causes profound, and sometimes prolonged, anterograde amnesia.

Indications
- Procedural sedation
- Sedation of an agitated or unco-operative patient prior to RSI
- Ongoing patient sedation post-intubation (often with an opioid)
- Reduction of side effects associated with ketamine.

Drug characteristics
- Onset over 2 minutes
- Plasma half-life is 2–6 hours, but the effects may be prolonged in elderly or debilitated patients
- Substantial variations in bioavailability have been reported.

Physiological effects
- Sedation
- Anterograde amnesia
- Respiratory depression
- Minimal cardiovascular depression (may cause bradycardia as well as hypotension)
- Vertigo and dizziness
- Visual disturbances and nausea.

Dose
- 0.02 to $0.08\,mg\,kg^{-1}$ IV usually achieves effective patient sedation.

Analgesia
Opioids

Although not recommended as part of the classic RSI technique, use of opioids will attenuate the cardiovascular responses to laryngoscopy and intubation. This may be particularly valuable if intracranial pressure is raised (see Trauma and raised intracranial pressure in Chapter 11), where the patient is very hypertensive or has ischaemic heart disease. Where opioids are used, the required dose of induction agent will be reduced.

Many opioids have a relatively slow onset of action. The respiratory depression caused by opioids may be troublesome if intubation fails, because the

Table 8.2. Commonly used opioids

	Alfentanil	Fentanyl	Morphine
Onset (minutes)	1	3	5
Duration (minutes)	10	40	180
Bolus dose	$10-20\,mcg\,kg^{-1}$	$1-3\,mcg\,kg^{-1}$	$100\,mcg\,kg^{-1}$
Physiological effects	Analgesia Respiratory depression Anaesthesia at higher doses	Analgesia Respiratory depression Anaesthesia at higher doses	Analgesia Respiratory depression
Main side effects	Muscle rigidity Bradycardia Hypotension	Muscle rigidity Bradycardia	Hypotension
Metabolism and excretion	Rapid liver metabolism	Liver metabolism	Renal clearance of active liver metabolites
Histamine release	No histamine release	Minimal histamine release	Significant histamine release

patient may remain apnoeic despite recovery from neuromuscular blockade; if necessary, reversal of the opioid with naloxone will restore spontaneous breathing. The effects of commonly used opioids are shown in Table 8.2.

Fentanyl is a potent synthetic opioid, which has a relatively fast onset (2–5 minutes) and short duration of action (30–60 minutes after a single dose). Its effects on the cardiovascular system are minimal, although large doses will cause bradycardia. Fentanyl (usual dose $1-3\,mcg\,kg^{-1}$ IV) will reduce the hypertensive response, and offset the increase in intracranial pressure caused by laryngoscopy and intubation, providing that two to three minutes have elapsed between giving the drug and intubation, but prolonged apnoea will also occur.

Alfentanil (usual dose $10-20\,mcg\,kg^{-1}$ IV) produces the same effects as fentanyl, but its peak action occurs after just 90 seconds and duration is 5–10 minutes: these characteristics make it ideal for attenuating the response to laryngoscopy and intubation.

If fentanyl or alfentanil are given, reduce the dose of induction drug.

Neuromuscular blocking drugs
Suxamethonium

Suxamethonium ($1.5-2\,mg\,kg^{-1}$) produces a dense neuromuscular block of rapid onset and short duration, making it the drug of choice for neuromuscular blockade during RSI. Initial depolarization at the neuromuscular junction causes muscle fasciculation within 15 seconds (although this is not always seen) and complete paralysis follows after 45–60 seconds. Spontaneous return of muscle activity follows after metabolism of the drug by plasma pseudocholinesterase.

Although it is the neuromuscular blocker of choice for rapid sequence induction, suxamethonium has significant side effects (see below).

Use
- Remains the first-line drug for muscular paralysis during rapid sequence induction.

Effects
- 10–15 seconds: fasciculations
- 45–60 seconds: paralysis
- 3–5 minutes: first return of respiratory activity
- 5–10 minutes: return of effective spontaneous ventilation.

Contra indications
- ECG changes suggesting hyperkalaemia
- Significant risk of hyperkalaemia: see Table 8.3.

Side effects
- Hyperkalaemia
- Bradycardia
- Fasciculation
- Muscle pain
- Histamine release
- Anaphylaxis
- Trigger drug for malignant hyperpyrexia in susceptible individuals
- Trismus/masseter spasm
- Prolonged neuromuscular blockade.

Dose
- 1.5–2 mg kg^{-1} IV.

Hyperkalaemia After injecting suxamethonium, the plasma potassium concentration is increased by up to 0.5 mmol l^{-1}, even in normal subjects. If the plasma potassium concentration is 6.0 mmol l^{-1} or higher the increase may precipitate arrhythmias, or even cardiac arrest. In addition, the increase in potassium concentration may be greatly exaggerated in patients with certain neurological diseases, particularly demyelinating conditions, desquamating skin conditions, major trauma, burns and several other pathologies. This can cause life-threatening hyperkalaemia. Although there are recognized periods of maximum risk for patients

Table 8.3. Pre-existing conditions in which suxamethonium may cause significant hyperkalaemia, and the periods of highest risk

Condition	Period of highest risk
Burns	2 days to 6 months
Peripheral neuropathy	5 days to 6 months
Spinal cord injury	5 days to 6 months
Upper motor neurone lesions or structural brain damage, including multiple sclerosis and stroke	5 days to 6 months
Muscular dystrophy	Continuing
Severe trauma, infection and certain skin conditions	Dependent on severity and duration

with these conditions (Table 8.3), the risks and benefits of using suxamethonium should be considered on an individual basis.

Bradycardia Suxamethonium may cause bradycardia, particularly if large or repeated doses are given: children are most at risk. This should be anticipated, and atropine must be available. Children do not need to be pre-treated with atropine routinely, but draw up the correct dose $(0.02 \, \text{mg kg}^{-1})$ and be ready to give it whenever a child is anaesthetized.

Muscle fasciculation The muscle fasciculations caused by suxamethonium can increase intracranial, intraocular and intragastric pressure. This effect is not significant when an adequate dose of an induction drug is given concurrently; therefore, pre-treatment with a de-fasciculating dose of a non-depolarizing drug is not necessary.

Muscle pain This is most likely to occur 12–24 hours after giving suxamethonium to fit young patients and those who mobilize quickly after anaesthesia. It is seldom a clinical problem in patients undergoing emergency anaesthesia.

Histamine release This will occur to a greater or lesser extent in all patients, and can cause significant hypotension.

Prolonged neuromuscular block With repeated doses of suxamethonium the characteristics of the neuromuscular block change, and paralysis may be prolonged. The action of suxamethonium may also be prolonged in the presence of organophosphate poisoning or cocaine use, when neuromuscular blockade may last 20–30 minutes. In patients with low or abnormal pseudocholinesterase activity, muscle paralysis after a dose of suxamethonium may last for several hours ('scoline' apnoea). Treatment for this condition involves continued ventilation (including sedation) until normal neuromuscular activity returns.

Table 8.4. Commonly used non-depolarizing neuromuscular blockers

	Atracurium besylate	Vecuronium bromide	Pancuronium bromide	Rocuronium bromide
Onset (minutes)	3–5	3–5	3–5	1
Duration (minutes)	20–35	20–35	60–90	30–60
Loading dose	0.3–0.5 mg kg^{-1}	0.05–0.1 mg kg^{-1}	0.05–0.1 mg kg^{-1}	0.6–1.0 mg kg^{-1}
Infusion rate	5–10 mcg kg^{-1} min^{-1}	1–2 mcg kg^{-1} min^{-1}	0.05–0.1 mg kg^{-1} hr^{-1}	0.1–0.5 mg kg^{-1} hr^{-1}
Metabolism/ excretion	Hofmann elimination	Hepatic/biliary	Hepatic/renal	Hepatic/renal
Notes	Histamine release: less accumulation	Cardio-stable	Increases heart rate	Rapid onset

Non-depolarizing muscle relaxants

In rare situations when suxamethonium is contraindicated, rocuronium $1.0\,mg\,kg^{-1}$ can be used for modified RSI, and will enable intubation after 60 seconds. This dose will cause paralysis for about an hour. Anaphylaxis to rocuronium occurs, but is less common than anaphylaxis to suxamethonium. A modified RSI using rocuronium instead of suxamethonium should be undertaken only by a practitioner with considerable experience.

Other non-depolarizing neuromuscular blockers are unlikely to be used during RSI, but may be used for maintaining muscle relaxation following recovery from suxamethonium. Commonly used non-depolarizing neuromuscular blockers are shown in Table 8.4.

Potential drug-related complications

The following complications can occur for the first time during emergency anaesthesia, but in some cases may be anticipated from the history of previous anaesthetics, allergies or family reactions to anaesthetic. This emphasizes the importance – even in emergencies – of thorough preparation, including a brief history where possible. Other information may also be found among the patient's possessions, wallet or MedicAlert jewellery.

Malignant hyperthermia

Malignant hyperthermia (MH) is a life-threatening disorder of skeletal muscle calcium homeostasis. Its inheritance is autosomal dominant, with an incidence of around 1 in 30,000. The most common triggers are suxamethonium and volatile anaesthetics. Diagnosis can be difficult, and it may present insidiously over hours or as an acute life-threatening event at induction. Hyperthermia itself may be a late feature, as are the effects of rhabdomyolysis. Signs can be considered in two groups: direct muscle effects and the effects of increased metabolism. Masseter muscle spasm (MMS) may indicate MH, and can be the only sign of it, but is not pathognomonic since it also occurs in a few normal patients, especially children, after suxamethonium. After injection of suxamethonium, MMS will cause trismus at a time when relaxation would normally have been expected, but it does not usually persist long enough to hinder attempts at intubation. Treat prolonged MMS as a potential case of MH.

The most common signs of increased metabolism are:

- unexplained increasing $ETCO_2$
- concomitant tachycardia and arrhythmias
- decreasing oxygen saturation
- flushing.

Having excluded ventilatory problems and light anaesthesia, a patient displaying these signs should be treated for MH.

The Association of Anaesthetists of Great Britain and Ireland have published guidelines for the recognition and treatment of malignant hyperthermia. These guidelines should be available wherever general anaesthesia is administered, and followed if MH is suspected. Seek senior anaesthetic assistance immediately in all cases of suspected MH.

Discontinue the precipitant and give dantrolene sodium as soon as the diagnosis is considered. The initial dose is 2.5 mg kg^{-1} IV, repeated every five minutes up to a maximum of 10 mg kg^{-1}. Dantrolene has no major side effects but reconstitution for injection is time-consuming; several people may be needed to help. Further treatment comprises: hyperventilation to reduce CO_2, increasing the FiO_2 to maintain adequate oxygenation of arterial blood, frequent monitoring of pH, arterial blood gases and potassium, and supportive therapy as required.

Anaphylaxis

Anaphylaxis is a severe, life-threatening, generalized or systemic hypersensitivity reaction. This is characterized by rapidly developing life-threatening airway and/or breathing and/or circulation problems usually associated with skin and mucosal changes. Almost any drug has the potential to cause one of these reactions. Other causes include contact with substances such as latex. The clinical manifestations vary but in the anaesthetized patient the incidences of various signs are:

- cardiovascular collapse 88%
- erythema 45%
- bronchospasm 36%
- angio-oedema 24%
- other cutaneous signs (swelling, urticaria, rash).

Anaphylaxis on induction will frequently present with acute cardiovascular collapse. The presence of severe bronchospasm may make ventilation of the lungs impossible, and acute upper airway oedema makes intubation difficult. In this situation a smaller tracheal tube or even a surgical airway may be necessary as other rescue devices such as the laryngeal mask airway will be relatively ineffective. A tension pneumothorax may also cause hypotension, high inspiratory pressures and desaturation of arterial blood, and should be considered, particularly in the trauma patient. If there is any doubt about the diagnosis, treat both conditions. Other diagnoses to consider are asthma, airway obstruction and primary myocardial pathology. The initial treatment of anaphylaxis is to remove the precipitant and to manage the airway, breathing and circulation:

- stop drug/remove precipitant
- 100% oxygen
- maintain airway
- get help
- lay patient flat with legs elevated
- adrenaline IV:
  - 50 mcg (0.5 ml of 1:10,000) increments (observing cardiac monitor) every 30 seconds until hypotension/bronchospasm improve
  - 1 mcg kg^{-1} in children = 0.1 ml kg^{-1} of 1:100,000

- 100–500 mcg or more may be required
- in severe cases consider an adrenaline infusion: the usual dose is 0.05–0.1 mcg kg^{-1} min^{-1}
- IV fluids – crystalloid (20 ml kg^{-1} in children).

Give antihistamines and corticosteroids to treat the end organ response to the mediators. A catecholamine infusion may be required as cardiovascular instability may last for hours. Check arterial blood gases regularly. Bronchodilators may be required to treat persistent bronchospasm. Before attempting extubation, ensure there is no residual oedema by deflating the tracheal tube cuff and checking for an adequate air leak.

- Antihistamines: chlorphenamine 10 mg slowly IV (0.25 mg kg^{-1} in children).
- Corticosteroids: hydrocortisone 200 mg IV (4 mg kg^{-1} in children).

The Resuscitation Council (UK) and The Association of Anaesthetists of Great Britain and Ireland have published guidelines for the recognition and treatment of anaphylaxis. These guidelines should be available wherever general anaesthesia is administered, and followed if anaphylaxis is suspected. Immediately seek senior assistance in all cases of suspected anaphylaxis.

Summary

- Knowledge of the pharmacology and side effects of drugs used commonly in emergency airway management is essential.
- No drug is perfect, and its advantages and disadvantages must be understood clearly.
- Practitioners should choose drugs with which they are most familiar.
- Practitioners must know how to treat the common complications of any drugs or techniques used.

Further reading

1 British National Formulary, Number 51. London: British Medical Association and the Royal Pharmaceutical Society of Great Britain, 2006.

2 Peck, T.E., Hill, S.A., Williams, M., Grice, A.S. & Aldington, D.S. (2003) *Pharmacology for Anaesthesia and Intensive Care*, 2nd edn. London: Greenwich Medical Media.

3 Association of Anaesthetists of Great Britain and Ireland (2004) Syringe labelling in critical care area (June 2004 update). London: Association of Anaesthetists of Great Britain and Ireland. See: www.aagbi.org/guidelines.html

4 Resuscitation Council (UK) (2008) Emergency treatment of anaphylactic reactions. London: Resuscitation Council (UK). See: www.resus.org.uk/pages/reaction.pdf

5 Association of anaesthetists of Great Britain and Ireland (2003) Anaphylactic reactions associated with anaesthesia 3 (revised 2003). London: Association of Anaesthetists of Great Britain and Ireland. See: www.aagbi.org/guidelines.html

6 Bergen, J.M. & Smith, D.C. (1997) A review of etomidate for rapid sequence intubation in the emergency department. *J Emerg Med*; **15**: 221–30.

7 Jackson, W.L. (2005) Should we use etomidate as an induction agent for endotracheal intubation in patients with septic shock? A critical appraisal. *Chest*; **127**: 1031–8.

8 Murray, H. & Marik, P.E. (2005) Etomidate for endotracheal intubation in sepsis: acknowledging the good while accepting the bad. *Chest*; **127**: 707–8.

9 Morris, C. & McAllister, C. (2005) Etomidate for emergency anaesthesia; mad, bad and dangerous to know? *Anaesthesia*; **60**(8): 737.

10 Kapklein, M.J. & Slonim, A.D. (2002) Ketamine v propofol: how safe is safe enough? *Crit Care Med*; **30**: 1384–6.

11 Rose, M. & Fisher, M. (2001) Rocuronium: high risk for anaphylaxis? *Br J Anaesth*; **86**: 678–82.

Difficult and failed airway

Dermot McKeown, Tim Parke and David Lockey

Objectives

The objectives of this chapter are to:

- understand the importance of maintaining oxygenation after failed intubation associated with rapid sequence induction (RSI)
- describe a plan for control of the airway and oxygenation after failed intubation
- understand the common causes of failure to obtain an adequate view of the larynx, and describe ways of improving the view
- understand the reasons for failure to intubate the trachea, and describe techniques that may improve success
- understand the techniques for rescue ventilation of the lungs.

At the conclusion of a planned RSI in a patient with an adequate circulation, failure to detect expired CO_2 indicates incorrect placement of the tracheal tube: under these circumstances the tube must be removed. Failure to place a tracheal tube correctly after an RSI is not a disaster, but failure to recognize incorrect placement, or to allow the patient to become injured during further attempts to secure an airway, are indefensible.

> If in doubt, take it out

Failed first attempt at tracheal intubation during RSI

This situation demands a logical sequence of treatment decisions: the urgency will be dictated by the rate of deterioration in the patient's physiology, which must be considered continuously during further treatment.

The fundamental questions are:

- Is the patient's arterial blood oxygenated enough to enable further attempts at intubation safely?
- If not, can it be improved?
- Were the intubating conditions ideal?
- Can the laryngeal view be improved?
- Can the intubation technique be improved?
- Should further attempts fail, are there suitable alternatives?
- Should further attempts fail, is a surgical airway necessary and possible?

Emergency Airway Management, eds. Jonathan Benger, Jerry Nolan and Mike Clancy.
Published by Cambridge University Press. © College of Emergency Medicine, London 2009.

Ensuring oxygenation

During airway interventions, constant attention must be paid to maintaining adequate oxygen saturation of the patient's arterial blood (SpO_2). No absolute rules for timing can be given, as the reserves of oxygen available to individual patients are variable: a previously fit young patient with a primary neurological problem, such as an isolated head injury, who has been carefully pre-oxygenated using a tight-fitting facemask, is likely to maintain a good SpO_2 during further intubation attempts; an obese patient with pulmonary contusions or pneumonia will desaturate rapidly without active ventilation with supplementary oxygen.

> Patients need oxygen, not a tube

Continuous SpO_2 monitoring is essential. Cease intubation attempts and re-oxygenate the patient's lungs before the decrease in SpO_2 reaches the steep part of the oxyhaemoglobin dissociation curve: this point is 92%. Delegate a member of the team to state when this point has been reached so that the practitioner will stop the intubation attempt and re-oxygenate the patient's lungs.

Oxygenation techniques

If the patient is still paralysed, bag-mask ventilation as described earlier is the first choice (see Chapter 4). Cricoid pressure is maintained initially, but if ventilation proves difficult, it should be reduced or gently released. Improvement in oxygenation is the main goal: this should be achieved easily if ventilation is efficient; even small volumes of high concentrations of oxygen can improve SpO_2 dramatically. At this stage effective oxygenation has priority over optimal ventilation and CO_2 removal.

To maximize the efficiency of bag-mask techniques, two practitioners are required: one to hold the mask and continue airway manipulations, and the other to ventilate the patient's lungs. Ideally, the second individual should also be experienced in airway management and ventilation. Use oropharyngeal and/or nasopharyngeal airways as necessary to improve airway patency.

If the SpO_2 continues to decrease despite optimal attempts at bag-mask ventilation, the first rescue technique of choice is to insert a laryngeal mask airway (LMA): this device should be familiar to all practitioners attempting intubation. The technique of insertion is described below. Several versions of the LMA are available but the most commonly encountered, and most widely used, is the standard device (classic LMA). In comparison with the classic LMA, the ProSeal LMA (PLMA) or intubating LMA (ILMA) have advantages and disadvantages; however, practice and familiarity with the standard device will assist in using the more advanced models.

Use of the laryngeal mask airway (LMA)

The LMA has transformed the airway management of patients undergoing elective surgery. If used correctly, it provides an excellent airway for the

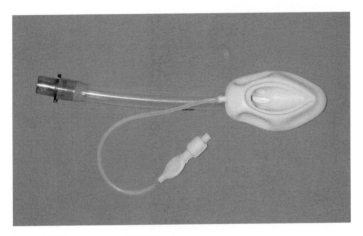

Figure 9.1 The laryngeal mask airway.

spontaneously breathing patient, and can also be used for controlled ventilation (Figure 9.1).

While it does not provide a cuffed tube in the trachea, and therefore is not considered a 'definitive airway', some degree of protection is afforded since a correctly placed LMA sits in the upper oesophagus and protects the glottic opening.

Laryngeal mask airways have also been used widely in emergency airway management. As rescue devices, successful insertion rates are high and they have several advantages over other failed airway techniques. Insertion skills are at least as easy to teach as for other devices, and are retained well.

The LMA is recommended as the rescue device of choice in the anaesthetic 'can't intubate, can't ventilate' (CICV) situation.

Developments of the classic LMA include the PLMA, which enables higher inflation pressures, drainage of the stomach via an oesophageal lumen, and probably greater protection against aspiration (Figure 9.2); and the ILMA, which enables blind passage of a specially designed tracheal tube. Blind intubation through the ILMA requires considerable practice before it can be achieved with consistently high success rates.

These will not be considered further, although the PLMA or other supra-glottic device may eventually become the preferred option for rescue ventilation. The recommended technique of insertion for each of these varies slightly from the original LMA; however, many experienced airway practitioners still prefer the original reusable device for emergencies.

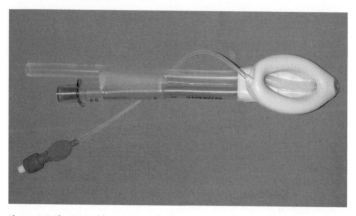

Figure 9.2 The ProSeal laryngeal mask airway.

Technique of insertion

- Remove the LMA from the packaging and lubricate the posterior surface with a water-soluble lubricant.
- Place an inflation syringe in the cuff valve, and deflate the cuff completely for insertion, ensuring that the leading tip is not folded backwards.
- Unless contraindicated, place the head and neck in the 'sniffing the morning air' intubation position.
- Open the mouth with a 'scissor' grip (in which the fingers and thumb cross), lifting the chin forward.
- Press the LMA against the hard palate, and guide it along the posterior oropharynx until it sits in position at the upper oesophagus. This technique minimizes the risk of the epiglottis folding downwards as the LMA is advanced.
- Remove the cricoid pressure during insertion to enable the LMA to sit correctly in the upper oesophagus.
- Inflate the cuff to $60\,cmH_2O$ (if a pressure device is available) or until a seal for ventilation is achieved (typically 20–30 ml for size 4 LMA and 30–40 ml for a size 5 LMA). Small movements of the mask may improve the seal and ventilatory efficiency.
- Fix the LMA in position with self-adhesive tape round the tube, and insert a bite-block.

If spontaneous respiratory effort resumes, assisted ventilation should be synchronized with breathing to minimize the leakage of gas from the larynx and risk of gastric distension. Insertion of the LMA is usually easy and improvement in ventilation rapid. Failure to achieve adequate ventilation may be caused by laryngospasm or obstruction from a folded-down epiglottis. If there is not rapid improvement, make a second attempt to place the LMA. Avoid repeated attempts at insertion if the patient's condition is deteriorating. If oxygenation cannot be maintained with an optimally placed LMA, a surgical approach to the airway is indicated (see below). Although this is a rare event, delay in recognizing the need for a surgical airway can be lethal.

Intubating conditions

Attempting intubation in the presence of muscle tone will cause problems: either failure to see the larynx because of gagging, or failure to pass the tracheal tube because of cord closure. Do not attempt laryngoscopy until the muscle relaxant is fully effective; for suxamethonium this is after the fasciculations have stopped. Loss of jaw tone will indicate the onset of relaxation. If conditions are not optimal, maintain oxygenation while awaiting muscle relaxation.

Manipulation of the tube can be difficult if it is soft (more likely if stored in warm conditions), or flexible because of small calibre. A malleable stylet may enable more efficient direction of the tube, but it will have to be removed if an intubating bougie is required. The stylet should never protrude from the distal end of the tracheal tube.

Do not use a tracheal tube that is too large for the larynx: it will make intubation much more difficult. A tube one or two sizes smaller must be available for immediate use, and the importance of skilled, dedicated assistance for the practitioner undertaking airway management cannot be over emphasized.

Can the laryngeal view be improved?

Although both parts of the RSI and intubation procedure, laryngoscopy and placement of the tube in the trachea can be considered as separate components. A full and clear view of the larynx will usually enable an 'easy' intubation; however, a single upper peg tooth can make placement of the tracheal tube difficult despite a good view and, very rarely, the patient may have an airway stenosis beyond the glottis. If the view at first attempt has been partially or totally obscured, there are several techniques that may improve the view. If preparation has been performed carefully, the first attempt should be the best.

> Always make the first attempt the best attempt

Improve the view by clearing secretions, blood and debris rapidly with a wide-bore suction device, followed by one or more of:
- head elevation
- external manipulation of the larynx
- use of an alternative laryngoscope blade
- change of practitioner.

Head elevation

Optimal positioning should have been achieved before the first attempt, but ensure that the head is extended fully at the atlanto-occipital joint and the neck is flexed. These manoeuvres cannot be applied to a patient whose cervical spine is stabilized. Hospital trolleys rarely have an adjustable head support, so insertion of a second pillow or doubling of the pillow may be necessary. An assistant lifting the head can be a suitable alternative, and may be combined with external manipulation of the larynx.

The obese patient poses considerable challenges, and careful positioning of the head and shoulders will facilitate intubation (see Figures 4.5 and 4.6).

Avoid 'levering' the laryngoscope, and ensure that the blade is lifted in the direction of the handle.

External manipulation of larynx

Manipulation of the larynx during laryngoscopy can improve the view: one technique is the **B**ackwards **U**pwards **R**ightwards **P**ressure (BURP) manoeuvre, which can be applied by an assistant. Alternatively, bimanual laryngoscopy has also been shown to be effective. In this technique the intubating practitioner initially applies external pressure over the thyroid cartilage with their right hand while simultaneously observing the view during direct laryngoscopy. Once the optimum view is achieved an assistant maintains this external laryngeal position, so that tracheal intubation can proceed. If necessary, the position can be modified during the procedure.

Use of an alternative laryngoscope blade

The practitioner should select their favoured blade from the outset – this minimizes the likelihood of needing to change the blade, particularly if a large blade is used. It may be reasonable to use the same blade again for a second attempt.

If the practitioner is familiar with alternative blades (and has maintained skills in their use) it is appropriate to change the blade once. A McCoy blade, with a hinged tip, is particularly useful where the epiglottis is long and floppy. Occasionally, lifting the epiglottis directly, rather than indirectly, will provide a view of the larynx. A straight blade, such as a Miller or Henderson type, requires a different technique, and needs practice to retain skills. An intubating bougie is often used with blades such as the Henderson, as insertion of the tube can otherwise be difficult even with a good view of the larynx.

Change of practitioner

As with any practical procedure, it is easy to become obsessed with the belief that 'I should successfully intubate this patient' rather than 'this patient should be successfully intubated'. If the first attempt has been the best attempt, and further manipulations have not been successful, another experienced practitioner may consider attempting intubation, but only if it is safe to do so. This must not result in a queue of potential experts performing multiple attempts; however, most series of emergency RSI failures demonstrate that a change of practitioner, particularly to a more experienced one, usually enables successful intubation. A change in practitioner also provides a useful educational opportunity to observe techniques that may prove successful.

This sequence may be conveniently remembered by the mnemonic **O HELP!**

O HELP!
- **O**xygenation
- **H**ead elevation
- **E**xternal laryngeal manipulation
- **L**aryngoscope blade change
- **P**al – call for assistance

If the second laryngoscopy fails to improve the view

If the view of the larynx cannot be improved, and oxygenation remains acceptable, an intubating bougie may be useful. Depending on their experience with this device, many practitioners use the intubating bougie at the initial laryngoscopy if the view is grade 2 or 3. This device can be passed into the trachea either anterior to visible arytenoids, where a grade 2 view is obtainable, or posterior to the epiglottis blindly if the view is grade 3. There may be a characteristic 'clicking' sensation appreciated as the angulated tip of the bougie moves over the tracheal rings, and there will be 'hold-up' detected as the tip enters the smaller bronchi. It is essential to advance the bougie gently, as excessive force can cause perforation of the airway. If muscle power is returning, there may be coughing or other reaction to tracheal placement of the bougie. Further information on the correct use of an intubating bougie is given in Chapter 7.

Several versions of the intubating bougie exist: the most reliable and preferred device is the Eschmann reusable tracheal tube introducer.

If repeat laryngoscopy fails, but oxygenation is maintained

In the 'can't intubate, can oxygenate' situation the practitioner must consider the following.
- Is spontaneous breathing present?
- Is ventilation adequate?
- Is the airway still at risk?
- Is intubation the only option at this time?

After a single dose of suxamethonium, in the absence of opioid, by the time that repeat laryngoscopy has been undertaken, intubation has not been achieved, and oxygenation is in progress, neuromuscular function is likely to be recovering and spontaneous breathing resuming. This should prompt synchronization of ventilatory assistance with spontaneous respiration, and a gradual return to the pre-RSI state.

Spontaneous breathing may be inadequate, and assistance may need to be continued to ensure either oxygenation, ventilation or both. Whether or not adequate spontaneous breathing has returned will dictate the need for, and urgency of, progression to alternative intubation techniques. A judgement of airway risk should also be made at this time: where oxygenation and ventilation are adequate, and airway patency is maintained, alternatives can be considered calmly; if the airway is deteriorating (e.g. expanding neck haematoma), there is far greater urgency. A choice must be made between continuing the intubation sequence, or accepting that the risk/benefit for this patient at this time is to cease intubation attempts and maintain the airway without intubation. If a 'best' attempt at laryngoscopy and intubation by an experienced practitioner has failed, and review of 'O HELP' has failed, it is unlikely that tracheal intubation will be achieved using standard methods.

> Patients do not die from failure to intubate, they die from failure to stop trying to intubate

This does not preclude further attempts using alternative techniques by experienced airway practitioners. Skills such as fibreoptic methods, retrograde techniques, and use of intubating laryngeal masks or light wands are difficult to acquire and retain, and beyond the remit of this manual (Box 9.1). The best option may be to maintain oxygenation and ventilation with basic techniques until an experienced practitioner arrives.

Box 9.1 Some alternative methods that may be used by expert practitioners

- intubating laryngeal mask with or without fibreoptic guidance
- alternative laryngoscopes (Bullard, Upsherscope, etc.)
- light-wand techniques
- fibreoptic laryngoscopy via laryngeal mask with Aintree catheter
- awake fibreoptic laryngoscopy and intubation
- retrograde intubation
- awake intubation with local anaesthesia
- blind nasal intubation
  This list is not comprehensive, and all techniques demand considerable practice to attain mastery.

If repeat laryngoscopy fails, and oxygenation is not maintained

The CICV situation is rare, but a logical plan must be in place to enable difficult decisions to be made rapidly. The first action is to insert an LMA. If oxygenation cannot be maintained with an LMA, consider the following questions.

- **Is a surgical airway necessary?**
- Are the patient's lungs being ventilated maximally with oxygen?
- **Is a surgical airway necessary?**
- Is arterial oxygenation stable and survivable? Can it be improved?
- **Is a surgical airway necessary?**
- Will a surgical airway be possible?
- Which form of surgical airway?

> The ideal rate of cricothyroidotomy is 100% in those who need it, and 0% in those who do not

Is a surgical airway necessary?
Creating a surgical airway is a rare event. Large case series in the US report cricothyroidotomy rates of 0.5% for emergency department intubations. This is considerably higher than the incidence in the UK and elsewhere in Europe. It is important to consider that a surgical airway may be necessary, and to be prepared to proceed: although early consideration is essential, it may not be mandated immediately.

Are the patient's lungs being ventilated maximally with oxygen?
If the patient's lungs are being ventilated adequately, yet oxygenation cannot be maintained at >90% SpO_2, check that oxygen is being delivered to the correct breathing system and to the patient. Disconnected tubing, failure to turn oxygen on and the use of other gases are all causes of oxygenation failure.

Is a surgical airway necessary?
Although the previous check has been rapid, the situation may be deteriorating. Failure to identify simple causes increases the likely need for a surgical airway.

Is arterial oxygenation stable and survivable? Can it be improved?
The SpO_2 in relation to the patient's pre-existing condition is important: a stable saturation of 85% in a patient with pulmonary oedema with apparently adequate ventilation may not be increased by intubation alone; application of positive end expiratory pressure (PEEP) or continuous positive airway pressure or bi-level positive airway pressure (CPAP/BiPAP) may slowly increase the SpO_2.

Stable, survivable oxygenation with no ventilatory difficulty and no impending airway problem is again a situation that may enable more experienced help to be mobilized.

Is a surgical airway necessary?
A surgical airway is indicated if a rapid check has shown no equipment problems and there is failure to ventilate and oxygenate the lungs.

Will a surgical airway be possible?
This is not the time to consider this. Assessment of the patient before RSI should have identified potential problems for individual patients. At this stage the

airway is required, and equipment must be immediately available. The team needs to be prepared and know their roles and responsibilities.

Techniques for rescue ventilation

Failure to intubate combined with failure to ventilate is an uncommon but time-critical situation, which occurs more commonly in victims of trauma. Rescue devices such as the classic LMA or one of its more recent variants may convert a 'can't ventilate' situation into a 'can ventilate' situation. If this fails a surgical airway or needle cricothyroidotomy are required. Published studies of emergency surgical airways demonstrate that, even in this stressful situation, success rates for this procedure are very high. The commonest error is performing the procedure too late, when hypoxaemic damage may have already occurred. There are various techniques that can be used, and many commercial kits are available. Doctors who may be responsible for emergency airway management must be familiar with the equipment in their hospitals and confident in its use. Most doctors will never have to perform a surgical airway, but if required to do so they must perform the procedure rapidly and effectively. The straightforward techniques described below require equipment that should be available in every emergency department.

Surgical cricothyroidotomy provides a definitive airway that can be used to ventilate the lungs until semi-elective intubation or tracheostomy is performed. Needle cricothyroidotomy is a much more temporary intervention providing only short-term oxygenation. It requires a high-pressure oxygen source, may cause barotrauma and can be particularly ineffective in patients with chest trauma. It is also prone to failure because of kinking of the cannula, and is unsuitable for maintaining oxygenation during patient transfer. It is often recommended in the (very rare) failed airway in a child, where surgical cricothyroidotomy is relatively contraindicated because of the risk of damaging the cricoid cartilage.

The final choice of surgical airway will depend upon the clinical situation, practitioner skills and experience. Options are:
- needle cricothyroidotomy
- surgical cricothyroidotomy
- tracheostomy.

Needle cricothyroidotomy

Insertion of a wide-bore, non-kinking cannula through the cricothyroid membrane and using this to deliver oxygen can be life-saving. The correct equipment must be available to connect to an oxygen source. This equipment should be identified clearly and stored for immediate use: an emergency is not the time to develop improvized solutions for oxygen delivery.

Experience with bench models of cricothyroid puncture may be useful and some practitioners will have experienced insertion of cannulae into the trachea during percutaneous tracheostomy. Needle cricothyroidotomy may not provide entirely adequate oxygenation and ventilation, and does not prevent the risk of aspiration, but will usually provide enough oxygenation to enable a more formal airway intervention to proceed.

Equipment required
- stiff cannula and needle (minimum 14 gauge in adults)
- syringe (preferably 20 ml)
- ventilation system that can be attached securely at one end to a high-pressure oxygen source at 400 kPa (4 bar), and at the other to the cannula. This should enable control of inspiration and expiration with effective pressure release.

Technique
- Attach the syringe to the rear of the cannula and needle assembly, and insert the cannula through the cricothyroid membrane into the airway at an angle of 45 degrees, aiming caudally in the midline. Confirm cannula position by aspiration of air with the syringe and advance the cannula fully over the needle into the trachea. Remove the needle, and aspirate air from the cannula to confirm position.
- Hold the cannula in place, attach the ventilation system and commence ventilation.
- One second of oxygen supplied at a pressure of 400 kPa (4 bar) and flow of 15 l min^{-1} should be sufficient to inflate adult lungs adequately. This is followed by a four-second pause to enable expiration via the upper airway (expiration does not occur via the cannula). In children, the initial oxygen flow rate in l min^{-1} should equal the child's age in years, and this is increased in 1 l min^{-1} increments until one second of oxygen flow causes the chest to rise.
- Look carefully for adequate exhalation through the upper airway. This usually occurs without difficulty, but it is essential to ensure that the chest falls adequately after each ventilation.
- If ventilation fails or complications occur, proceed immediately to surgical cricothyroidotomy.

Note: a major problem with this technique is occlusion of the cannula after insertion. This is especially likely where a soft, kinkable intravenous cannula is used.

Surgical cricothyroidotomy

The cricothyroid membrane is relatively avascular and normally easy to feel. Extension of the neck (if possible) will improve surgical access and exposure.

Equipment required
- scalpel (preferably 20 blade: rounded rather than pointed)
- 6 or 7 mm cuffed tracheal tube
- tracheal dilator (artery clip if unavailable).

Technique
- Rapidly but accurately identify the cricothyroid membrane.
- Make a horizontal stab incision through the membrane into the airway.

- Open the incision with tracheal dilators (with the scalpel blade still *in situ*).
- Remove the scalpel blade and insert the tube. Inflate the cuff and confirm tube position.

Note: this procedure should be completed in approximately 30 seconds.

Be careful not to damage the posterior tracheal wall by deep penetration with the scalpel blade. If the incision is too small to admit the tube the incision can be enlarged laterally while being held open vertically with the tracheal dilator. Ideally, once a passage is made into the trachea it should be occupied by instruments until a tube is inserted. This technique prevents loss of the passage at a crucial time and minimizes bleeding. A tracheal tube is preferred to a tracheostomy tube because the cuff of a small tracheostomy tube is often too small to occlude an adult trachea.

Tracheostomy

A surgical tracheostomy will rarely be indicated as a primary method of securing the airway. This is a formal surgical procedure that cannot be undertaken safely without training. Percutaneous tracheostomy can be used in emergencies, but only by individuals experienced in the single-stage dilatational approach.

Summary

- A well planned RSI by an experienced practitioner with adequate pre-assessment will have a high success rate for correct placement of a tracheal tube at the first attempt.
- If the tube is not inserted easily, and oxygenation is well maintained, several rapid manipulations may be made in an attempt to improve the laryngeal view and optimize intubating conditions.
- If intubation is still unsuccessful, ensure adequate oxygenation before a second laryngoscopy and intubation sequence. This attempt may include repositioning, external laryngeal manipulation, and a change of equipment or practitioner. An intubating bougie will frequently be used to assist intubation with reduced view (grade 2 or 3).
- Failure to intubate again must be followed by re-oxygenation/ventilation, and a reassessment of the need and urgency for intubation.
- The rescue technique of choice is bag-mask ventilation, but if this fails insert an LMA.
- Adequate oxygenation and ventilation and a stable airway at this point will enable careful consideration of a different approach by a practitioner with specialist airway skills.
- Continued failure to oxygenate mandates rapid checks for remediable causes.
- If oxygenation continues to deteriorate, a surgical airway is indicated. The method chosen will depend on patient and practitioner factors.

Further reading

1 Henderson, J.J., Popat, M.T., Latto, I.P. & Pearce, A.C. (2004) Difficult Airway Society guidelines for management of the unanticipated difficult intubation. *Anaesthesia*; **59**: 675–94.

2 American Society of Anesthesiologists Task Force on Management of the Difficult Airway (2003) Practice guidelines for management of the difficult airway. An updated report. *Anesthesiology*; **95**: 1269–77.

3 Levitan, R.M. (2003) Patient safety in emergency airway management and rapid sequence intubation: metaphorical lessons from skydiving. *Ann Emerg Med*; **42**: 81–7.

4 Murphy, M.F. (2003) Bringing the larynx into view: a piece of the puzzle. *Ann Emerg Med*; **41**: 338–41.

5 Levitan, R.M., Kinkle, W.C., Levin, W.J. & Everett, W.W. (2006) Laryngeal view during laryngoscopy: a randomised trial comparing cricoid pressure, backward-upward-rightward pressure, and bimanual laryngoscopy. *Ann Emerg Med*; **47**: 548–55.

6 Bair, A.E., Panacek, E.A., Wisner, D.H., Bales, R. & Sakles, J.C. (2003) Cricothyrotomy: a 5-year experience at one institution. *J Emerg Med*; **24**: 151–6.

7 The Difficult Airway Society of the United Kingdom. This medical society was formed in 1995 and aims to improve management of the patient's airway by anaesthetists and critical care personnel. Website and algorithms are available at: www.das.uk.com

Post-intubation management and preparation for transfer

Paul Younge, David Lockey and Alasdair Gray

Objectives

The objectives of this chapter are to:

- understand the principles of patient management following successful intubation
- understand the principles of monitoring, ongoing sedation and neuromuscular blockade for intubated patients
- be familiar with the correct operation of transport ventilators
- be familiar with the principles of patient preparation for safe transfer.

Introduction

After a successful rapid sequence induction (RSI) has been performed there is often an understandable sense of relief that the airway has been secured. However, intubation is only the initial phase of management; the post-intubation phase is equally important.

Following emergency airway management, most patients will need transfer to other areas such as the radiology department, intensive care unit (ICU), operating theatres or tertiary care in another hospital. The key questions are:

- What is the predicted clinical course?
- Is the patient stable enough to transfer?
- Is any further treatment required?

The objectives of the post-intubation phase are to achieve enough physiological stability for transfer, and to carry out other appropriate treatment.

The requirements for stabilization and the nature of treatment may vary considerably: for example, a patient intubated for overdose can often be stabilized and treated while waiting for an ICU bed. A patient with a suspected traumatic extradural haemorrhage should undergo CT scanning as soon as adequate physiological stability is achieved. An unstable multi-trauma patient may need urgent transfer to the operating room to achieve surgical haemorrhage control.

This phase can be described using a modified ABCDE system. The sections below form a checklist. While an ABCDE system suggests progress in a consecutive manner, procedures will normally be carried out simultaneously when a team is involved.

Emergency Airway Management, eds. Jonathan Benger, Jerry Nolan and Mike Clancy.
Published by Cambridge University Press. © College of Emergency Medicine, London 2009.

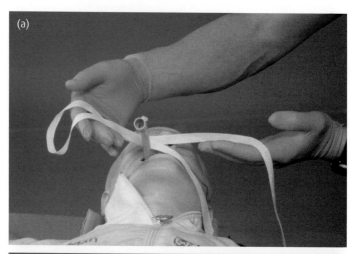

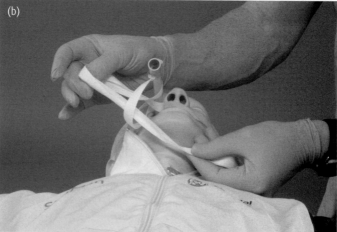

Figure 10.1 *Method of securely tying the tracheal tube in position* (a) A loop of ribbon is made above the tracheal tube: the two free ends should be of different lengths so the final knot is located away from the midline. (b) Both ends of the ribbon are passed through the loop, forming a 'slip knot' around the tracheal tube: this automatically tightens as tension is applied. (c) The two ends of ribbon are separated, and the loop is pulled tight around the tube. (d) The two ends of the ribbon are passed in opposite directions around the patient's neck, and secured away from the midline with an appropriate knot.

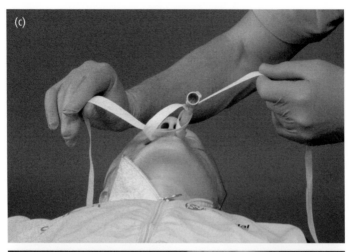

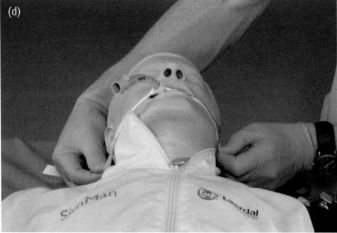

Figure 10.1 (*cont.*)

Airway

Is the airway secure?

Secure the tracheal tube at the correct length with a tie or tape to avoid unplanned extubation, or intubation of the right main bronchus. There are many methods of securing a tracheal tube: choose one that is safe, effective and familiar. A common method for tying the tube is shown in Figure 10.1.

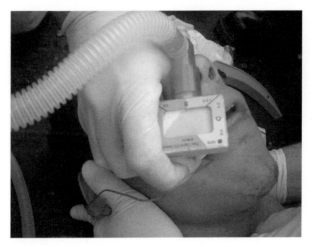

Figure 10.2 Colourimetric CO_2 detector in use.

Tape is sometimes preferred in the setting of head injury to avoid encircling the neck and impeding venous return, which may increase intracranial pressure. Several commercial fixation devices are also available. These are effective but rather more expensive than the conventional alternatives.

Has end tidal CO_2 monitoring been attached?
A simple disposable qualitative colourimetric device (Figure 10.2) can be used to detect the presence of exhaled CO_2 and confirm correct tracheal tube placement (e.g. yellow for 'yes', purple for 'poor'). However, continuous quantitative end tidal carbon dioxide ($ETCO_2$) measurement enables monitoring of alveolar ventilation and respiratory pattern. It is particularly important in the setting of head injury where precise control of $PaCO_2$ is required. Record the $ETCO_2$ at the time an arterial blood sample is taken: this enables calibration of the $ETCO_2$ against $PaCO_2$. The latter may be significantly higher because of V/Q mismatch.

Is the cervical spine adequately stabilized?

Is an HME (heat and moisture exchanger) at the patient end of the circuit?
Apart from protecting equipment from contamination this will help keep the patient warm and maintain airway humidification. This prevents excessive drying of secretions and reduces the rate of respiratory infection.

Breathing

Is ventilation satisfactory?

This is mainly assessed clinically, based on chest expansion and breath sounds, but is augmented by pulse oximetry, $ETCO_2$ measurement and arterial blood gas analyses.

Initially, the patient's lungs are ventilated manually, which enables an assessment of chest compliance and assists in the detection of any respiratory obstruction. If possible, the patient is then transferred to a portable ventilator: this gives constant ventilatory support and helps achieve a steady state. Check arterial blood gases when mechanical ventilation is commenced and 20 minutes later to guide adjustment of ventilator settings.

Patients with very stiff lungs, such as those with pulmonary oedema, or with a prolonged expiratory phase, such as those with severe asthma, may need hand ventilation until a ventilator of higher specification is available.

Ventilator settings will depend initially on clinical assessment of chest expansion. A brief guide to the features of a transport ventilator is given below. Use manufacturer's instructions and your medical physics or anaesthetic technical services department to instruct you on your particular ventilator.

In some modes of ventilation the ventilator does not interact with a patient's efforts to breathe, while in others it detects and interacts with those efforts. Controlled mandatory ventilation (CMV) is the most commonly used non-interactive mode in the emergency setting. A respiratory rate and tidal volume are set to determine a minute volume. Synchronized intermittent mandatory ventilation (SIMV) enables the patient to initiate ventilator breaths. Where a patient does not initiate breaths the set SIMV breath rate is delivered in the same way as CMV ventilation (giving a back-up minute volume). This is useful if neuromuscular blocking drugs have not been given, if the patient has recovered from neuromuscular blockade, or if weaning or assessing the presence of respiratory effort. Regular suction of secretions is also important.

Transport ventilators

See Figures 10.3 and 10.4. All transport ventilators have a CMV mode. Some also have SIMV, and can deliver CPAP, and others also have a pressure control ventilation mode.

Some less sophisticated transport ventilators deliver a set minute volume (MV) that is divided into a number of breaths per minute (respiratory rate (RR)). A disadvantage of this is that decreasing the RR without altering MV will increase the tidal volume (V_T) and ventilation pressures. A peak airway pressure-limiting (P_{max}) valve must be incorporated to protect against this. Later models have controls for V_T and RR to overcome this problem as well as pressure-limiting valves and alarms. A disconnect alarm should be standard, but is not present on all transport ventilators: models without an integral disconnection alarm must be watched very carefully because they will continue to cycle even if there is no patient attached. Simpler models have a fixed inspiratory:expiratory (I:E) ratio of 1:2.

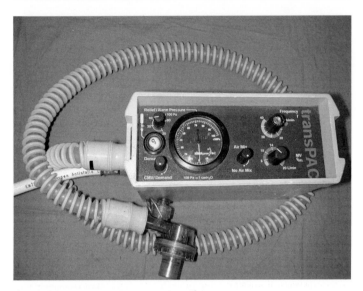

Figure 10.3 Pneupac transPAC transport ventilator.

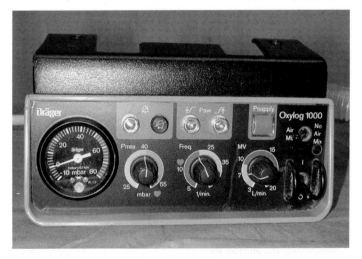

Figure 10.4 Dräger Oxylog 1000 transport ventilator.

Table 10.1. Ventilator troubleshooting

Problem	Solution
Not ventilating: no noise or pressure	Check on/off (I/O) switch
	Check O_2 source/connections
Not ventilating: noise but no pressure generated	Check for disconnections
	Check ventilation valve
	Check for tracheal cuff leak
Not ventilating: noise and pressure generated	Check for kinks or obstruction in the tubing
	Patient may be fighting the ventilator
	Patient may have stiff lungs
	Check for tension pneumothorax

Others enable selection of I:E ratios over a wider range. Inspired oxygen concentration (FiO_2) is normally 100% or 60% (air mix).

Use of some degree of positive end expiratory pressure (PEEP) is recommended in most patients. If a simple transport ventilator does not have this capacity, a PEEP valve can be attached at the patient end of the circuit.

Before attaching to the patient perform a quick ventilator check.

- Connect O_2 supply via a Schraeder valve to the wall supply or cylinder.
- For a 'standard' adult set FiO_2 to 1.0 by switching to 'no air mix' or selecting 100% oxygen. Set RR to 12, MV to 6 litres and the P_{max} to 40 cmH$_2$O.
- Connect to a test 'lung' (or use the reservoir bag of an anaesthetic breathing system).
- Switch the ventilator on and check that the 'lung' inflates and deflates.
- Squeeze the 'lung' to simulate obstruction or increasing airway pressures and check that the P_{max} alarm sounds.
- Disconnect the circuit and check that the disconnect alarm sounds. Note that the alarm is silenced for about two minutes by pressing the silence button.

When connected to the patient it is best to set a rate (RR) then gradually increase the MV until an adequate tidal volume is achieved clinically.

Obtain another chest X-ray to check the position of the tracheal and nasogastric tubes.

Has a naso- or orogastric tube been placed?
Insertion of a tube into the stomach enables deflation of a dilated stomach and removal of stomach contents. This helps to reduce the potential for aspiration and may sometimes enable lower ventilation pressures. It also enables diagnosis of haemorrhage and provides access to the gastro-intestinal (GI) tract for treatments such as activated charcoal.

Are chest drains required?

Chest trauma, particularly rib fractures, is associated with pneumothoraces. Small pneumothoraces may not be visible on chest X-ray, especially if they are anterior, and a tension pneumothorax may develop from a simple pneumothorax. This is a particular risk when positive pressure ventilation is commenced. Prophylactic chest drains may be inserted, particularly if the patient is about to be transported or undergo a lengthy procedure when the chest will not be immediately accessible. If a chest drain is not inserted then careful monitoring is essential, with rapid intervention to drain the chest if there is any evidence of a developing pneumothorax.

Circulation

Decisions about the use of fluids and/or inotropes will depend on the diagnosis. Clinical assessment, which includes capillary refill time and urine output, is most important. An arterial line is considered standard if the patient is haemodynamically unstable or at risk of becoming unstable. A central venous catheter may guide fluid therapy and provide venous access, but should not delay urgent transfers.

In most cases, it is appropriate to maintain a mean arterial pressure of 70 mmHg or more and a CVP of greater than 12 mmHg. Exceptions to this include:

- penetrating injury or uncontained haemorrhage, when hypotensive resuscitation may be appropriate
- head injury – when it is judged that a higher mean arterial pressure (typically 90 mmHg) is required to maintain an adequate cerebral perfusion pressure.

Hypotension

- Exclude hypovolaemia.
- All anaesthetic drugs can cause hypotension – adequate intravascular volume is required before and after induction. If induction causes hypotension, fluids and vasopressor drugs may be required.
- Exclude tension pneumothorax.
- Excessive PEEP may cause hypotension, particularly if there is pre-existing myocardial impairment.
- Record a 12-lead ECG.

Hypertension

Usually indicates inadequate analgesia or sedation unless associated with severe head injury, or raised intracranial pressure from other causes.

Disability

Check the adequacy of:

- sedation
- analgesia
- paralysis
- seizure control.

Sedation and analgesia

Sedation techniques vary: usually, a sedative drug is combined with an opioid. Propofol infusions are convenient and used in a wide variety of clinical situations. Anticonvulsant properties make it suitable for head injury or status epilepticus; it is also a bronchodilator and therefore useful for patients with asthma. It should be used carefully in patients with hypovolaemia. The concurrent use of opioids reduces the dose of propofol required to maintain adequate sedation.

Midazolam is an alternative sedative drug. It has more cardiovascular stability, and is often combined with morphine or fentanyl. The advantage of these drugs is that they can be given by bolus, which may be useful during transport. Remifentanil, an ultra short acting opioid, has recently been introduced, and is increasingly used in some ICUs; it is expensive.

Muscle relaxation

In many situations it is appropriate to paralyse intubated patients. This is particularly important for transfers. The risk of extubation is reduced, ventilation is facilitated and sudden increases in intracranial pressure caused by gagging are avoided. Vecuronium and atracurium are suitable drugs: the properties of these and two other commonly used drugs are summarized in Table 8.4.

Seizure control

Seizures are controlled in the normal way with benzodiazepines such as lorazepam or diazepam. Propofol or midazolam are also effective anticonvulsants. It is common practice to give a loading dose of phenytoin after a second seizure.

Exposure and environment

The exposure required for the secondary survey, combined with the vasodilatory effects of anaesthetic drugs, may cause significant cooling. This is generally harmful except in those who have been resuscitated from cardiac arrest, and possibly patients with head injuries.

Temperature should be monitored and warming blankets used where appropriate; warmed fluids and warmed humidified oxygen are also effective.

Transfer to definitive management

Intubated patients in the emergency department will usually require transfer from the resuscitation room to another department in the hospital, or to another hospital for continuing care. It is not always possible for the patient to be physiological stable before transfer. For example, the patient may require transfer directly to the operating theatre for laparotomy after completion of the primary survey. However, the patient should be as stable as possible before transfer. Common destinations include the CT scanner, operating room and ICU in the same hospital, and specialist centres such as neurosurgery in other hospitals.

During transfer the patient is at significant risk of adverse events and these are associated with worse outcome. Many of these adverse events are avoidable if

---

Box 10.1 Checklist for transfer

- Airway safe. Tube position confirmed by end tidal CO_2 monitoring and chest X-ray.
- Patient paralysed, sedated and ventilated.
- Adequate gas exchange confirmed by arterial blood gas (ABG).
- Chest tubes secured, where applicable. (Heimlich valve preferred to underwater seal.)
- Circulation stable, haemorrhage controlled.
- Abdominal injuries properly assessed and treated.
- Minimum of two routes of venous access.
- Adequate haemoglobin concentration.
- Seizures controlled.
- Long bone and pelvic fractures stabilized.
- Temperature maintained.
- Acid–base, glucose and metabolic abnormalities corrected.
- Case notes, X-rays and transfer documentation.
- Cross-matched blood with the patient, if appropriate.
- Appropriate equipment and drugs. All devices compatible with ambulance equipment. Spare batteries. Sufficient oxygen supplies for the journey (see Box 10.2).
- Communication with receiving clinicians.

---

attention is paid to the preparation of the patient before transfer. A checklist for transfer appears in Box 10.1.

Preparation

Preparation should follow the system described in previous sections of this chapter.

Personnel

An appropriately trained person who is aware of the risks of transportation should attend an intubated patient at all times. They should have specific training in the transportation of the critically ill. Ideally, a specialist retrieval team should transport children as this reduces critical incidents. Accompanying staff transferring patients between hospitals should have high visibility protective and warm clothing and a means of communicating with the hospital, i.e. a mobile phone. They should be insured for injury and have an identified method of returning to their base hospital.

Equipment

All equipment used during transport should be reliable, portable and robust. Accompanying staff should be familiar with the equipment. Battery life should

---

Box 10.2 Calculating the oxygen required for patient transfer

Oxygen calculation:
$2 \times$ transport time in minutes $\times [(MV \times FiO_2) +$ ventilator driving gas$]$
Give yourself at least one hour of extra O_2.
FiO_2 is a proportion e.g. $60\% = 0.6$.
Ventilator driving gas varies, but is commonly $1 \, l \, min^{-1}$.
e.g. for MV of $10 \, l \, min^{-1}$ at an FiO_2 of 0.6 over a one-hour trip:
O_2 required $= 2 \times 60 \times [(10 \times 0.6) + 1] = 840 \, l =$ two 'E' or one 'F' oxygen cylinder.
Note: one 'E' cylinder at $15 \, l \, min^{-1}$ flow will last only 45 minutes.

---

be long enough for transfer or an alternative should be easily available, such as an adapter to connect to the ambulance power source. Oxygen requirements need to be calculated. The recommended formula is described in Box 10.2.

During transport equipment should be secured and not lying free on the patient. An equipment bridge mounted over the patient and attached to the transport trolley, or a specially designed transport trolley, are ideal. These must be compatible with local ambulance service equipment. Physiological parameters, including pulse, invasive blood pressure, oxygen saturation and quantitative end tidal CO_2, should be visible to the clinician at all times on a multiple parameter transport monitor. The ability to measure central venous pressures and core temperature should also be available. A transport bag or rucksack complete with emergency drugs, fluids and airway equipment should be carried during transfer.

Documentation

Review and update the clinical records. Record observations regularly, usually at 15-minute intervals. The standard of observation should be the same as in an ICU throughout the assessment and resuscitation period, and during transfer. Outstanding investigations should be organized and results reviewed and documented. Complete a pre-transfer checklist before transfer. Ensure that all relevant documentation, including drug charts, fluid charts and copies of investigations such as X-rays go with the patient. In some cases cross-matched blood will also be required.

Communication

There should be clear communication between all clinical specialties involved in the patient's care. If referral or care is discussed via the telephone, document this communication clearly in the clinical records. This should include the names of the clinicians and the time and date. The receiving department should be aware of the departure of the patient from the resuscitation room. For example, the CT scanner should be free and available *before* the patient leaves the emergency department. A receiving hospital should also receive adequate warning of the patient's arrival. If the accompanying staff have not been involved in the patient's care before transfer, adequate handover must take place before transportation. Speak to the patient's relatives before transfer to definitive care. Give them directions to the receiving hospital department and inform them who they should speak to. There should be a recognized method for contacting the local ambulance service and ensuring rapid availability of a fully equipped ambulance for transfer. Ambulance personnel must know the location of the receiving hospital and department before transfer. Discuss with ambulance personnel the urgency of the transfer and requirement for 'blue lights'.

Considerations during transport

The patient is most at risk when they are being moved; for example, transfer into the CT scanner or from the resuscitation room to the ambulance. At this time there is a significant possibility of the tracheal tube or intravascular access being dislodged. Careful co-ordination and attention to detail during these manoeuvres will reduce the likelihood of these events happening. Handover and transfer to the bed at the receiving department is also a time of risk and the patient should be settled and all monitoring, drug infusions and ventilation transferred and continued before formal handover occurs.

If preparation has been thorough there should be little to do during transport, apart from continuous monitoring of the patient. Ensure that monitors are clearly visible and intravascular access secured and accessible at all times. Prepare drugs that may be required during transfer before departure; label them and ensure that they are immediately accessible to the accompanying staff. The aim is for no intervention to be necessary during transport. If the patient requires attention during transfer, stop the ambulance. Document and review any critical incidents that occur.

Summary
- The post-intubation phase is an integral part of emergency airway management.
- The objectives of the post-intubation phase are to achieve enough physiological stability for transfer, and to carry out other appropriate treatment.
- A modified ABCDE system provides useful prompts to correct and complete patient management.
- Practitioners must be familiar with the drugs and equipment commonly used in the post-intubation phase.
- Thorough and systematic preparation is essential for safe patient transfer.

Further reading

1 Association of Anaesthetists of Great Britain and Ireland (2000) *Recommendations for Standards of Monitoring*, 3rd edn. London: Association of Anaesthetists of Great Britain and Ireland. See: www.aagbi.org/guidelines.html

2 Intensive Care Society (2002) *Standards and Guidelines: Transport of the Critically Ill Adult.* London: Intensive Care Society.

3 Association of Anaesthetists of Great Britain and Ireland (2006) *Recommendations for the Safe Transfer of Patients with Brain Injury.* London: Association of Anaesthetists of Great Britain and Ireland.

Emergency airway management in special circumstances

Patricia Weir, Paul Younge, Andy Eynon, Patrick Nee, Alasdair Gray, Dermot McKeown, Neil Robinson, Carl Gwinnutt, David Lockey and Jonathan Benger

PAEDIATRICS
Objectives
The objectives of this section are to:
- understand the principles of emergency airway management that apply to children
- understand the key airway differences between adults and children
- appreciate the need to obtain early specialist help with paediatric airway management.

Introduction
The need to intubate children in an emergency using drugs outside an operating theatre is rare. Even in very busy centres this will occur only around once a month. It is therefore difficult to obtain and maintain the necessary skills. In most institutions skilled airway assistance in the form of an experienced anaesthetist will be available quickly and their help should always be sought.

Do not attempt RSI in children unless:
(a) You have appropriate skills and training, OR;
(b) In an emergency – when the patient's airway, and adequate oxygenation, cannot be maintained using basic airway manoeuvres such as an oropharyngeal airway and bag-mask ventilation, and assistance is **not imminent**

Special considerations in children
Anatomical
See Figure 11.1.
- Head size (large occiput) – causes neck flexion.
- The infant's tongue is relatively large in proportion to the rest of the oral cavity. It therefore more easily obstructs the airway, and is more difficult to manipulate with a laryngoscope blade.

Emergency Airway Management, eds. Jonathan Benger, Jerry Nolan and Mike Clancy.
Published by Cambridge University Press. © College of Emergency Medicine, London 2009.

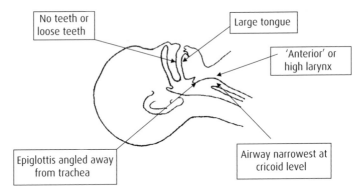

No teeth or loose teeth

Large tongue

'Anterior' or high larynx

Epiglottis angled away from trachea

Airway narrowest at cricoid level

Figure 11.1 Anatomical features of a child's airway that differ from an adult.

- The infant's larynx is higher in the neck (C3–4) than in an adult (C4–5).
- The epiglottis is angled away from the axis of the trachea, and it is therefore more difficult to lift the epiglottis with the tip of a laryngoscope blade.
- The narrowest portion of the infant larynx is the cricoid cartilage (compared to the vocal cords in an adult). Therefore a tracheal tube will pass through the cords and be tightly wedged against the tracheal wall at the level of the cricoid, causing damage to the tracheal mucosa and potential sub-glottic stenosis or post-extubation stridor.
- The trachea is relatively short, increasing the risk of bronchial intubation or extubation during patient transfer.
- No teeth in infancy.

The child develops adult anatomy by the age of 10–12 years. The greatest anatomical differences exist in the infant (i.e. <1 year).

Physiological
- High basal oxygen consumption (6 ml kg^{-1} min^{-1}, or twice that of adults).
- Lower functional residual capacity (FRC).
- Children therefore have significantly less oxygen reserve, and will desaturate much faster than adults (Figure 2.11).

Drugs
- Drug dosage. The effective doses of induction drugs such as propofol and thiopental sodium are relatively greater in children of 6 months to 16 years (Table 11.1).

> Ensure an adequate dose of suxamethonium! Remember to have a follow-up dose of a non-depolarizing neuromuscular blocker drawn up to give once the airway is secure (e.g. vecuronium 0.1 mg kg^{-1}, atracurium 0.6 mg kg^{-1})

Table 11.1. Drug doses for induction and neuromuscular blockade in children

Induction	Stable child	Propofol 2.5–3 mg kg^{-1}, or, thiopental sodium 3–5 mg kg^{-1}
	Unstable child	Ketamine 2 mg kg^{-1} and fentanyl 2 mcg kg^{-1}, or, midazolam 0.1 mg kg^{-1}
Neuromuscular blockers	Weight < 20 kg	Suxamethonium^a 2 mg kg^{-1}, flushed with normal saline
	Weight > 20 kg	Suxamethonium 1–2 mg kg^{-1}

Note:
^{a}Fasciculation is not seen in young children.

- Pre-treatment with anticholinergics is not undertaken routinely. However, always give atropine 0.02 mg kg^{-1} before a second dose of suxamethonium, and ensure that the correct dose of atropine is drawn up and ready to give before RSI is undertaken in children.

Cricoid pressure
The application of cricoid pressure in neonates and young infants (< 6 months) is controversial. If applied poorly, it may distort the larynx resulting in a poor or no view of the vocal cords. Therefore, some clinicians advocate not applying it in this age group. If cricoid pressure is applied and the larynx is not seen then the practitioner should either ask the assistant to let go, or should undertake external laryngeal manipulation to improve the view.

Position
Positioning will be age dependent because of the anatomical considerations outlined above. The optimal position for intubation is the same as for bag-mask ventilation (Table 11.2).

There is a tendency for the infant head to roll from side to side; this can be controlled by the use of a sandbag, fluid bag or towel at the side of the head.

Equipment
Oropharyngeal airways
These are available from size 000 (absolutely tiny and rarely required) to adult size.

Sizing of oropharyngeal airways is important as too small an airway will get buried in the tongue, and too large an airway may hit and push down the

Table 11.2. Optimal patient positioning for effective airway management in children of various ages

Pre-term/ex-prem	May require a small roll under shoulders to compensate for large occiput.
Infant (up to 1 year)	Neutral position – because of the large occiput naturally resulting in neck flexion.
Small child (<8 years)	Head tilt, chin lift resulting in neck flexion/head extension.
Older child (> 8 years)	With increasing age a small pillow may need to be put under the child's head to achieve optimal conditions.

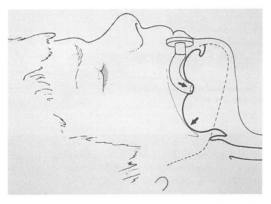

Figure 11.2 Position of an oropharyngeal airway that is too short.

epiglottis (Figures 11.2 and 11.3). Measurement from the incisor teeth to the angle of the jaw will give approximately the correct size. If the child appears to be swallowing the airway, it is too small, and if it fails to seat fully in the mouth, it is too big. The technique for insertion in children is the same as for adults, but rough manipulation will cause trauma. In infants the airway should be inserted the correct way up (i.e. the way that it will ultimately sit), using a laryngoscope blade or a tongue depressor to facilitate placement.

Facemasks

Clear plastic cuffed facemasks enable good contour fit onto the face, and detection of colour change or vomit.

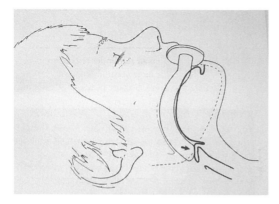

Figure 11.3 Position of an oropharyngeal airway that is too long.

Suction
Yankauer Must be available, connected and functioning at induction.

Narrow-bore Should be available for immediate use once the tracheal tube is in position. The correct size in French gauge (FG) is twice the diameter of the tracheal tube (i.e. an 8 FG suction catheter will fit down a size 4.0 mm tracheal tube).

Breathing systems
Self-inflating bags These are safe and easy to use; there are many types, but they are generally manufactured in three sizes – neonatal (approx. 250 ml), child (approx. 500 ml) and adult. Neonatal bags may not produce sufficient tidal volumes when used in non-neonates, especially if there is a poor seal around the facemask. Therefore their use should be restricted to neonatal units only.

Most self-inflating bags designed for children have a pressure relief valve set at around 45 cmH₂O. This can be overridden if required by placing a finger on the valve. It is not usually necessary to do this; however, if it is deemed necessary to override the valve, consider the potentially reversible causes of high airway resistance such as obstruction or blockage in the breathing system or tension pneumothorax.

Ayres T-piece These require experience and a fresh gas source to use, but are popular with anaesthetists as they enable assessment of lung compliance and the ability to switch from IPPV to spontaneous ventilation with ease. These systems are generally single patient use and available with 500 ml or 1 litre bags.

Sufficient fresh gas flow (FGF) is required when using an Ayres T-piece to avoid or minimize rebreathing of expired CO_2.

For spontaneous ventilation: FGF = 2–3 × minute ventilation
For IPPV: FGF = 1000 ml + 200 ml kg^{-1}

Laryngoscopes

Differences in the anatomy of the larynx in infants (i.e. <1 year) make a straight-bladed laryngoscope the instrument of choice in this age group. This is placed beneath the epiglottis and lifted to expose the larynx.

Straight-bladed laryngoscopes are narrower and preferred by many anaesthetists for children under five years, as they allow more room in the mouth; alternatively, a size 2 Macintosh (curved blade) can be used in this age group.

Tracheal tubes

A non-cuffed tracheal tube is used in the pre-pubertal child to minimize damage to the tracheal mucosa. The correct size in children over one year can be calculated using the formula:

Internal diameter of the tracheal tube = [Age in years / 4] + 4

The 0.5 mm size above and below should always be available. Term babies will generally require a 3.5 mm tracheal tube.

In elective surgery, it is optimal to have a slight leak of air around the tracheal tube when applying 20 cmH$_2$O pressure: this ensures that the tube is not tightly wedged against the tracheal mucosa. However, in an emergency, there is often decreased lung compliance and it may be necessary to use a tube half a size larger to prevent excessive leak.

There is no consensus on whether or not a tracheal tube should be cut. In an emergency it is better to have a longer tracheal tube, which can be repositioned if required, than a tracheal tube that subsequently proves to be too short and may fall out.

Stylets and bougies

Stylets are generally stiff wire covered in plastic, designed to stiffen the tracheal tube and enable it to be angled towards the larynx. They have the potential to cause significant trauma, and must not protrude from the distal end of the tracheal tube. Stylets are particularly useful when inserting small tracheal tubes (4.0 mm or less), which lack intrinsic rigidity. Inexperienced practitioners may find it easier to routinely mount a stylet in smaller tracheal tubes before commencing intubation.

Bougies are designed for use in difficult intubations: they are inserted into the trachea enabling a tracheal tube to be railroaded into position. Orange/red paediatric bougies are available in several sizes: these are stiffer and potentially more traumatic than the traditional adult intubating bougie.

Before use, it is imperative to check that the tracheal tube fits over a chosen bougie, and that it is well lubricated.

Rapid sequence induction technique in children
Pre-oxygenation

Children must be pre-oxygenated as well as possible because their oxygen reserve is less and their arterial blood will desaturate quickly (Figure 2.11). The ideal is at least three minutes breathing 100% oxygen; however, this can be difficult to achieve in an unco-operative child. During elective anaesthesia, pre-oxygenation can be achieved by encouraging the child to take three to four maximal inspiratory breaths.

Ideally, pre-oxygenation should be carried out with a breathing system that can deliver 100% oxygen and has a low resistance to breathing, such as an Ayres T-piece. Pre-oxygenation with a self-inflating bag and mask in infants requires considerable effort; avoid it unless there is no other option.

Position patient appropriately for age and size (see above).

Equipment – have you got everything? (Box 11.1)

Box 11.1 Equipment for intubation

- Facemask
- Breathing system
- Oropharyngeal airways
- Yankauer suction catheter
- Laryngoscope
- Tracheal tubes
- Paediatric Magill's forceps
- Fine-bore suction catheters
- Nasogastric tube
- Tape/ties
- $ETCO_2$ measurement

Laryngoscopy

A reproducible technique for intubating neonates and small infants is to introduce the laryngoscope from the right and move to the centre, ensuring the blade is in the midline. Move down over the tongue and epiglottis, past the larynx, then gently pull back until the larynx falls into view.

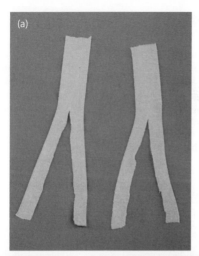

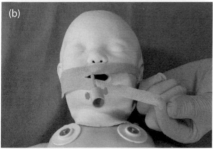

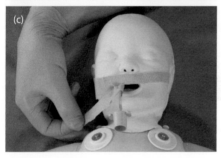

Figure 11.4 *Elastoplast fixation of the tracheal tube in children.* (a) Two pieces of Elastoplast tape, cut ready for use. (b) Take the first piece and attach the uncut end to the right cheek. With a bit of stretch on the tape put the upper limb across the upper lip. (c) Wind the lower limb securely around the tracheal tube.

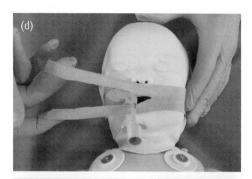

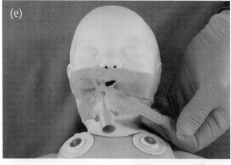

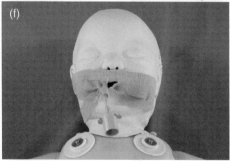

Caption for Figure 11.4 (*cont.*) (d) Take the second piece and attach the uncut end to the left cheek. (e) Stretch the lower limb and place this across the lower lip, then wind the upper limb securely around the tracheal tube. (f) Tracheal tube taped securely in position.

In older children the tip of the laryngoscope blade can be placed in the valecula (as for adults), lifting in the line of the handle to expose the vocal cords.

Insert the tracheal tube and check for chest movement, leak and presence of $ETCO_2$, and bilateral equal air entry on auscultation.

It is easy to insert the tracheal tube too far in small children, which usually results in passage into the right main bronchus

Fixation of the tracheal tube

There are many ways to fix tracheal tubes, including commercial fixation devices. In children, taping is preferable to tying and a simple and effective method is to use one-inch pink 'Elastoplast trouserlegs' (Figure 11.4).

Take the first piece and attach the uncut end to the right cheek. With a bit of stretch on the tape put the upper limb across the upper lip, then wind the lower limb securely around the tracheal tube. Take the second piece and attach it to the left cheek. Take the lower limb and place this across the lower lip, then wind the upper limb around the tracheal tube.

If the patient is going to be transported, provide additional stability by inserting an oropharyngeal airway and applying a third piece of Elastoplast with a central hole cut to accommodate the tracheal tube.

The difficult airway in children

Difficult airways are uncommon in normal children, but they do occur in association with acute upper airway obstruction and craniofacial anomalies (e.g. Pierre Robin, Goldenhar's, etc.). These can usually be anticipated by observation of the child's facial features or clinical status. If a difficult airway is anticipated, seek senior anaesthetic help. Seek help early in acute upper airway obstruction, or in syndromic children.

Summary

- There are significant differences between adults and children. Do not attempt RSI and tracheal intubation in young children unless you have appropriate training and experience. Always seek the help of an experienced paediatric anaesthetist.
- Children desaturate quickly: pre-oxygenate as thoroughly as possible.
- Check that you have *all* the correct equipment for children before commencing RSI and tracheal intubation.

Further reading

1 Advanced Life Support Group (2005) *Advanced Paediatric Life Support. The Practical Approach*, 4th edn. London: BMJ Books/Blackwells.
2 Carwell, M. & Walker, R. W. M. (2003) Management of the difficult paediatric airway. *Contin Educ Anaesth Crit Care Pain*; **3**: 167–70.

TRAUMA AND RAISED INTRACRANIAL PRESSURE (ICP)

Objectives

The objectives of this section are to:

- understand the importance of emergency airway management in minimizing secondary brain injury
- understand the importance of extracranial injuries in the resuscitation of patients with traumatic brain injury (TBI)
- understand the principles of safe transfer of trauma patients.

Introduction

In the UK, trauma remains the commonest cause of death in the first four decades of life. The Advanced trauma life support (ATLS©) programme stresses the importance of rapid assessment of trauma victims with simultaneous resuscitation of the airway (with cervical spine control), breathing and circulation (with haemorrhage control). A brief conversation with the patient will provide important information about airway patency, adequacy of breathing and circulation, and a rough estimate of the Glasgow Coma Scale (GCS) score. High-flow oxygen is applied immediately via a mask with a reservoir bag. In the first minute a decision is made about immediate, urgent or observant management of the airway (see Chapter 5). If the patient is in the immediate or urgent categories, a plan is made for intubation, with consideration of the drugs to be used and an additional 'plan B', to be followed if problems such as failed airway occur.

Airway

In the trauma patient, the airway may be compromised by:

- secretions, vomit, blood
- foreign body
- burns, smoke inhalation
- maxillofacial injuries
- depressed conscious level
- blunt or penetrating injury to the neck.

Airway management will depend on the urgency of intubation, the experience of the practitioner, the ability to get experienced help quickly and the equipment available.

Rapid sequence induction is indicated in trauma and head injury in the following circumstances:

- failure of the patient to maintain their own airway
- inadequate spontaneous breathing
- depressed conscious level
- anticipated deterioration in airway, breathing or conscious level
- before transfer in some cases.

Cervical spine management

Cervical spine injury (CSI) is assumed in all major trauma victims and patients with moderate or severe head injury. Stabilize the cervical spine with a rigid cervical collar, head blocks and tapes, or by using in-line manual stabilization. Clinical decision rules have been developed to assist in ruling out CSI, but these can be applied only to patients who are alert and co-operative. Early cervical spine clearance is impossible when the patient is obtunded, and the whole spine must be protected from uncontrolled movement until further investigations are completed.

Patients are removed from a spine board as soon as possible after arrival in the emergency department. Immobilization on a firm mattress is sufficient for the management of spinal injuries. Transfer to the imaging suite or other centre is facilitated by using a patient slide and vacuum mattress.

Orotracheal intubation using RSI is the technique of choice in head-injured patients, and those at risk of CSI. The hard collar, head blocks and tape are removed, and replaced with manual in-line stabilization provided by a designated assistant. This person stands or kneels at the side of the patient, either above or below the head, to allow the airway practitioner unimpeded access (Figure 11.5).

Cervical spine stabilization from above the head is common when intubating on a trolley in hospital, because the assistant can kneel to the left-hand side of the intubating practitioner, causing minimal obstruction. Out of hospital, or where patients are intubated lying on the ground, it is sometimes more expedient to stabilize the cervical spine from below the head. This gives the assistant a better view and causes less obstruction to the intubating practitioner. However, this technique reduces access to the neck, and it is important to ensure that full mouth opening is not prevented by holding the head too low.

In an alert patient significant force is required to exacerbate a cervical spine injury, because the spine is protected by muscle spasm. Once induction drugs and neuromuscular blockers have been given the cervical spine is more at risk. The assistant providing neck stabilization should therefore indicate immediately if any movement is detected during intubation.

Record in the notes the methods used to protect the patient from further spinal injury.

Rapid sequence induction in trauma and traumatic brain injury

Rapid sequence induction enables optimum oxygenation and ventilation to protect the injured brain from secondary insult, and facilitates further investigation and transfer.

The technique of RSI is described in Chapters 6 and 7. A difficult airway must be anticipated in trauma, and techniques for this are described in Chapter 9.

Secondary insults must be minimized during RSI. Intravenous induction drugs are indicated even in obtunded patients, because effective sedation and analgesia limits the increase in ICP associated with laryngoscopy and intubation. Consider pre-treatment with fentanyl or alfentanil (see Chapter 8) to reduce the sympathetic response to intubation.

There is no ideal induction drug, and practitioners should choose drugs with which they are most familiar, modifying the dose according to the patient's condition. Sodium thiopental and propofol have cerebroprotective effects, reducing

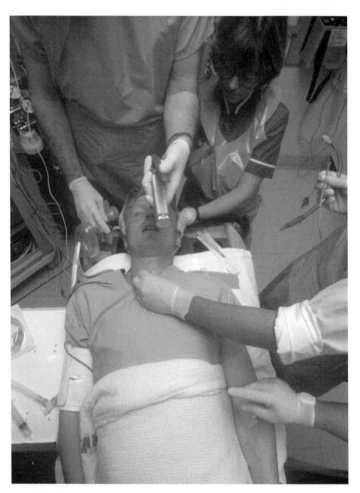

Figure 11.5 Manual in-line cervical spine stabilization during intubation.

the cerebral metabolic rate for oxygen ($CMRO_2$) and cerebral blood flow, thus reducing ICP; however, they can cause profound hypotension. Ketamine has sympathomimetic and vagolytic actions that may be useful when an increase in heart rate is desired, but it also increases the $CMRO_2$, and may increase intracranial pressure. Ketamine is therefore relatively contraindicated in TBI. Etomidate causes less cardiovascular depression than thiopental or propofol; however, it causes adrenal suppression, even after a single dose, and this may be clinically significant in the subsequent care of some patients.

When given with an adequate dose of an induction drug, suxamethonium does not cause a significant increase in ICP, and its rapid onset of action makes it the first choice neuromuscular blocker in TBI.

> Use the drugs with which you are most familiar, but remember that considerable dose reduction may be required in critically ill and injured patients

Breathing

Look for evidence of a tension pneumothorax, open pneumothorax or massive haemothorax and treat these immediately. Flail chest, pulmonary contusions, multiple rib fractures and simple pneumothorax all reduce the respiratory reserve. With major chest injuries, even 100% oxygen may fail to oxygenate the patient adequately and rapid desaturation is likely if drugs are given to facilitate intubation. Positive pressure ventilation can convert a simple pneumothorax into a tension pneumothorax. Consider placing chest drains before transfer in intubated patients with small pneumothoraces and/or multiple rib fractures. If a chest drain is not placed then careful communication and monitoring is required, including a clear plan to intervene immediately if there are signs of tension pneumothorax.

Ventilator settings require adjustment in trauma victims, especially those with chest trauma who are particularly at risk of acute respiratory distress syndrome (ARDS). Historically, the lungs of most patients were ventilated with high tidal volumes of at least $10 \, \text{ml kg}^{-1}$ with the aim of maintaining a normal $PaCO_2$. This can cause ventilator associated lung injury (VALI) from overdistension of alveoli (volutrauma), repeated recruitment and collapse of alveoli, and high pressure induced damage (barotrauma). Ventilation with lower tidal volumes (around 6–$8 \, \text{ml kg}^{-1}$ ideal body weight) and limiting plateau pressure increases survival in patients with ARDS. However, hypercarbia must be avoided in TBI patients because of the risk of raised ICP.

Circulation

All trauma victims are likely to have overt or covert blood loss. Signs of shock may be hidden, especially in children and young adults. Tachycardia does not always occur in hypovolaemia, and cardiac pacemakers and the use of drugs such as beta-blockers may also influence the heart rate. It is essential that reliable venous access is secured and that fluid resuscitation is established early. Circulatory insufficiency may also have non-haemorrhagic causes such as tension pneumothorax, cardiac tamponade, myocardial contusion or neurogenic shock. Intravenous fluid infusion is the appropriate initial treatment for circulatory shock in trauma, regardless of the underlying cause.

Table 11.3. Causes of secondary brain injury

Intracranial	Extracranial
Haematoma	Hypoxaemia
Cerebral oedema	Arterial hypotension
Seizures	Hypercarbia
Vasospasm	Hypocarbia
Infection	Anaemia
Hydrocephalus	Pyrexia
	Hyponatraemia
	Hypoglycaemia
	Hyperglycaemia

Anaesthetic induction drugs are vasodilators. Many practitioners recommend having adrenaline or noradrenaline to hand, although this does not reduce the need for adequate venous access and volume resuscitation.

Neurological injury

Traumatic brain injury is divided into primary and secondary brain injury. Primary injuries are caused by mechanical disruption to the brain occurring at the time of the initial trauma (contusion, laceration, diffuse axonal injury). Secondary injuries are subdivided into intracranial and extracranial causes (Table 11.3). Forty per cent of patients with severe TBI also have another significant extracranial injury. The severity and duration of hypoxaemia (SaO_2 less than 90%) or hypotension (systolic blood pressure less than 90 mmHg) adversely affect mortality. The principal treatment aim is to prevent secondary injuries and preserve the potential for neurological recovery.

Raised ICP and reduced cerebral perfusion pressure (CPP) also increase mortality. Raised ICP is common in patients with an abnormal CT scan and persisting coma after resuscitation, and in patients over 40 years with a normal CT scan but abnormal posturing and prior episodes of arterial hypotension. Hypoxaemia, hypercarbia and hypotension are the commonest causes of raised ICP in the absence of a haematoma, and these insults must be anticipated and treated promptly. Early intubation is required in all cases of coma-inducing TBI, and should be considered in patients with lesser degrees of impaired conscious level in association with extracranial injuries or agitation.

The relationship between mean arterial blood pressure (MAP), ICP and cerebral perfusion pressure (CPP) is set out below. By convention the impact of the central venous pressure (CVP), which also counters CPP, is ignored. The normal ICP is 0–10 mmHg. Traumatic brain injury patients with GCS less than 9 are likely to have an ICP of at least 20–30 mmHg. Regional hypoperfusion of the injured brain may occur when the CPP falls below 60 mmHg. It is therefore essential to maintain a MAP of at least 90 mmHg with fluids, inotropes, vasoactive drugs and careful selection and use of sedative and analgesic drugs. A MAP of 90 mmHg may be too high for polytrauma victims with ongoing haemorrhage: every effort should be made to control the haemorrhage and minimize secondary brain injury.

$$CPP = MAP - ICP$$

Post-intubation management

Once the patient has been intubated, mechanical ventilation is instituted. Sedation, with or without paralysis, relieves distress and enables effective control of oxygenation and ventilation. The ventilator is set to ensure that oxygen saturation remains above 98% and PaO_2 greater than 12 kPa. Hyperventilation may reduce cerebral perfusion, and $PaCO_2$ should not be reduced below 4.5 kPa. Avoid high positive end expiratory pressure (PEEP) and maximum inspiratory pressure (P_{max}) because these will reduce venous return from the head, causing venous congestion of the brain.

A continuous infusion of an intravenous anaesthetic and an opioid are used to maintain sedation and analgesia. The commonest combinations are propofol and fentanyl or alfentanil, or midazolam and morphine. Propofol and fentanyl/alfentanil are shorter acting and enable faster recovery of consciousness when discontinued. Midazolam and morphine can be given by bolus and may be preferred during transport.

Routine use of neuromuscular blockade varies between different centres. If the patient is to remain paralysed for some time, an IV infusion of a neuromuscular blocker such as atracurium or vecuronium can be used. Intermittent boluses of neuromuscular blocker are discouraged because coughing or gagging on the tracheal tube will increase ICP. Long-term use of neuromuscular blockers, especially the aminosteriods (such as rocuronium and vecuronium), is associated with the development of critical care neuromyopathy.

Transport and monitoring

In patients intubated for trauma and TBI the minimum monitoring requirements are:

- ECG
- SpO_2
- $ETCO_2$, with frequent validation against arterial blood gases
- intra-arterial pressure monitoring
- central venous pressure
- tympanic or other form of central temperature measurement. Recorded frequently: disordered thermo-regulation is relatively common.

The level of sedation, muscle relaxation, GCS, pupil size and pupil reactivity are recorded at least every 15 minutes. Strict fluid balance charts are maintained, with euvolaemia the target. Insert orogastric and urinary catheters in all patients.

The principles of safe preparation for transfer are described in Chapter 10. These should be followed closely, whether the patient is transferred within the hospital (CT scan, angiography suite, operating theatre, intensive care unit (ICU)) or to a specialist unit in another hospital. Deterioration in physiological status is common during transportation, and this has an adverse effect on outcome.

The agitated patient

Agitation after trauma may have one or more causes including hypoxaemia, shock, head injury, intoxication, pain and anxiety. Agitation must be controlled so that the patient can be properly assessed and managed without causing further injury to themselves or others. Always assume that the patient has a potentially life-threatening condition, and not that they are merely intoxicated. Sedation may be achieved using intravenous midazolam, but only to facilitate the process of RSI. Use small, incremental doses of 1–3 mg and allow time for the drug to act before administering further doses. In some cases RSI may be performed to facilitate subsequent CT scanning, and it may be appropriate to wake the patient after the scan, and when any other urgent investigations and procedures have been completed.

Summary

- Adequate resuscitation, with avoidance of hypoxaemia, hypercarbia and arterial hypotension, improves outcome in major trauma and TBI.
- Rapid sequence induction is the technique of choice for securing the airway: it is essential to have a 'plan B' if this fails.
- Always assume the presence of a cervical spine injury.
- All patients with major trauma have reduced physiological reserve: careful selection of drugs and dosages is required.

Further reading

1 Association of Anaesthetists of Great Britain and Ireland (2006) *Recommendations for the Safe Transfer of Patients with Brain Injury*. London: Association of Anaesthetists of Great Britain and Ireland.

2 Yentis, S. M. (1990) Suxamethonium and hyperkalaemia. *Anaesth Intensive Care*; **1**: 92–101.

3 National Institute for Health and Clinical Excellence (2003) *Head Injury – Triage, Assessment, Investigation and Early Management of Head Injury in Infants, Children and Adults*. London: National Institute for Health and Clinical Excellence. Available at: www.nice.org.uk/page.aspx?o=56817

4 Krantz, B., Ali, J., Aprahamian, C. *et al.* (2004) *Advanced Trauma Life Support Course Provider Manual*, 7th edn. Chicago: American College of Surgeons.

5 Kendall, R. & Menon, D. K. (2002) Acute head injury: initial resuscitation and transfer. *Anaesth Intensive Care Med*; **3**: 131–5.

6 British Trauma Society (2003) Guidelines for the initial management and assessment of spinal injury. *Injury*; **34**: 405–25.

CARDIORESPIRATORY FAILURE
Objective
The objective of this section is to:
- describe the indications, risks and technique for the intubation of patients with severe cardiorespiratory disease.

Introduction
Respiratory and cardiovascular emergencies are common indications for intubation in the emergency department. These patients generally require intubation because of failure to maintain adequate oxygenation and/or ventilation. Patients in extremis may need intubating for airway protection. The intubation process is identical to that described in Chapter 7.

Rapid sequence induction and intubation of patients with severe respiratory and/or cardiovascular disease is hazardous, with a greatly increased risk of complications during and after intubation. A reduced cardiac output and slower circulation time prolongs the onset and exaggerates the effects of drugs; i.e. there is increased sensitivity to the cardiorespiratory depressant effects of induction drugs. These patients have a low FRC and therefore reduced oxygen reserve. Mechanical ventilation has a significant effect on the heart and lungs, including a reduction in venous return leading to a decreased cardiac output, and the risk of lung injury caused by high inspiratory volumes.

Rapidly obtain as much information as possible about the patient's past medical history and social circumstances before intubation; this may include information from hospital records, GP, relatives and carers. Many of these patients have acute exacerbations of a pre-existing illness, such as chronic obstructive pulmonary disease or chronic heart failure, or may be elderly with multiple co-morbidities. Admission to an ICU may not be appropriate for some of these patients and, whenever possible, early assessment by an intensivist is desirable.

Consider alternatives to intubation and ventilation, such as non-invasive ventilatory support. This is discussed further in Chapter 12. However, if intubation is indicated and significant collateral history is not available, the patient must be fully resuscitated immediately while awaiting further information.

Respiratory emergencies
Asthma
Indications for intubation Consider intubation and invasive ventilation in any patient with asthma who is tiring, or where gas exchange continues to deteriorate (decreasing PaO_2 or increasing $PaCO_2$) despite optimal medical management. Follow the guidelines on the management of asthma published jointly by the British Thoracic Society (BTS) and Scottish Intercollegiate Guidelines Network (SIGN). All patients who have signs or symptoms of life-threatening asthma may potentially need intubation, especially those who have required

ventilatory support before. Refer to the intensivist team if any of the following are present, even if intubation is not required immediately:

- deteriorating peak expiratory flow
- persisting or worsening hypoxaemia
- hypercapnia
- arterial blood gas analysis showing a worsening acidaemia
- exhaustion, feeble respiration
- drowsiness, confusion
- coma or respiratory arrest.

Standard therapy includes high-flow oxygen via a facemask with reservoir bag, continuous beta$_2$ agonist and an anticholinergic drug such as ipratropium by nebulizer, oral or intravenous steroids and intravenous magnesium.

Specific considerations during intubation The patient will potentially be very difficult to pre-oxygenate because of hyperexpansion and reduced ventilatory capacity. A reduced oxygen reserve makes the asthmatic patient prone to hypoxaemia during intubation. Give a rapid infusion of fluid before and during induction of anaesthesia: patients with acute severe asthma will be dehydrated. Stimulation of the larynx and trachea can provoke laryngospasm and bronchospasm. Once the tube has been placed in the trachea initiate ventilation carefully, with gentle inspiration and a long expiratory phase as the already hyperexpanded lung is vulnerable to further expansion and volutrauma.

Ketamine Ketamine is a potent bronchodilator and an alternative to the standard induction drugs in patients with asthma. It has a relatively rapid onset intravenously: a dose of 1.5–2 mg kg^{-1} IV is used for induction. Peak concentrations are reached after one minute, and last for 10–15 minutes.

Use ketamine with caution in patients with ischaemic heart disease or hypertension, as it causes catecholamine release. It may also cause increased airway secretions, activation of pharyngeal reflexes and laryngospasm. Emergence phenomena are not usually a clinical problem in the emergency setting, but can be minimized with a small dose of benzodiazepine.

Post-intubation care There are several specific considerations in the treatment of an asthmatic patient after intubation.

The expiratory airflow obstruction that occurs in patients with severe asthma may cause air trapping, evidenced by high airway pressures, and lung hyperinflation. This will generate significant intrinsic positive end expiratory pressure (PEEP$_i$ or auto-PEEP) and over-distension of alveoli, which increases intra-thoracic pressure, reduces venous return and cardiac output, and causes hypotension. If this occurs, immediately disconnect the ventilator tubing from the tracheal tube and wait for complete exhalation: slow, steady chest compression may help to achieve adequate exhalation. The hypotension associated with auto-PEEP is exacerbated by hypovolaemia, which emphasizes the importance of fluid resuscitation before and immediately after RSI and intubation. Auto-PEEP is minimized by setting the ventilator to deliver the lowest minute volume that maintains oxygenation, and by providing a long expiratory time: providing the pH is above approximately 7.15 (H^+ 71 nmol l^{-1}) hypercarbia (permissive hypercapnia) is normally well tolerated. Asthmatic patients are at significant risk of developing tension pneumothoraces: these require immediate decompression. Any pneumothorax, whether under tension or not, will require insertion of a chest drain.

A bolus of a neuromuscular blocker such as vecuronium may be required to prevent the patient fighting the ventilator and further increasing airway pressure. Ensure that sedation is adequate. The addition of opioids will reduce respiratory drive, and are particularly useful when a strategy of permissive hypercapnia is used.

Mucous plugging occurs commonly in severe asthma: large plugs can occlude the tracheal tube, making it very difficult to ventilate the patient's lungs, and mucous plugging of the more distal airways can cause atelectasis, impairment of gas exchange and increased airway pressure. Therapeutic bronchoscopy may be necessary to remove large mucous plugs.

Chronic obstructive pulmonary disease (COPD)
The management principles for RSI and intubation of patients with COPD are similar to those with asthma.

Indications for intubation Careful consideration as to whether invasive ventilation is appropriate should be made by a senior clinician, and ideally by the patient's respiratory specialist. Consider alternatives to IPPV, such as non-invasive ventilatory support, which reduces the need for intubation (see Chapter 12). Patients with COPD may require intubation if they are unable to clear secretions, protect their airway, continue to deteriorate despite non-invasive ventilatory support and medical therapy, or become apnoeic. The BTS suggests that IPPV should be instituted in patients who have an explicit remedial cause for their deterioration (e.g. pneumonia, or the first episode of respiratory failure) and an acceptable quality of life. Age and the $PaCO_2$ level should not be used in isolation to determine whether intubation is appropriate.

Considerations during intubation By the time that patients with COPD require intubation they are often exhausted, have little oxygen reserve and are usually hypovolaemic. This makes them liable to arrhythmias and hypotension after intubation. A patient with COPD will require fluid loading and a reduced dose of induction drug for intubation. Normal doses of muscle relaxant are appropriate.

Post-intubation care The potential complications and difficulties of positive pressure ventilation are the same for patients with COPD as they are for those with asthma.

Cardiovascular emergencies
Acute cardiogenic pulmonary oedema

Acute cardiogenic pulmonary oedema with respiratory failure is a relatively common medical emergency in the UK. The average UK emergency department will see between 50 and 100 of these patients per annum and, despite medical therapy and non-invasive ventilation, 5–7.5% will require intubation. Medical therapy includes high-flow oxygen via a mask with a reservoir bag, sublingual, buccal or intravenous nitrates, and consideration of intravenous loop diuretics. Continuous positive airway pressure (CPAP) is frequently effective: see Chapter 12.

Cardiogenic shock

These patients are critically ill and at significant risk of complications including cardiac arrest immediately after induction. It is often necessary to support the circulation before intubation with intravenous fluids and/or careful use of vasoactive drugs. If there is concomitant pulmonary oedema it may be difficult or impossible to pre-oxygenate adequately; furthermore, any induction drug may reduce cardiac output catastrophically. A carefully selected small dose of induction drug should be used, and may have to be omitted completely in patients in extremis; in these circumstances a small dose of midazolam (0.5–1 mg) will provide adequate sedation and amnesia for the intubation. In these patients, the circulation time for drugs is very prolonged. After intubation, avoid over ventilation because this will reduce venous return and cardiac output.

Dissection of the thoracic aorta or rupture of an abdominal aortic aneurysm

Unless absolutely necessary, avoid intubating patients with vascular emergencies such as dissection of the thoracic aorta or rupture of an abdominal aortic aneurysm. Intubation is best accomplished in the operating room with a scrubbed surgical team standing by. During intubation, the aim is to ablate the physiological response to laryngoscopy and intubation, and to prevent surges in blood pressure and heart rate. A pre-induction dose of an opioid such as fentanyl or alfentanil will reduce the sympathetic stimulation caused by laryngoscopy and intubation. Fentanyl is effective only if it is given at least three minutes before intubation, but be prepared to progress to intubation immediately if the patient becomes apnoeic.

Cardioversion

Patients who are physiologically compromised, or have significant symptoms such as chest pain, with either a broad- or narrow-complex tachycardia may require electrical cardioversion. The initial management of these arrhythmias should follow European Resuscitation Council guidelines on peri-arrest arrhythmias. Electrical cardioversion is painful and therefore requires analgesia and sedation. There is no consensus on the best drugs to provide sedation or anaesthesia for cardioversion. Possibilities include carefully titrated doses of midazolam, propofol or etomidate; any of these can be combined with a short-acting opioid such as fentanyl or alfentanil.

These drugs provide a brief period of analgesia, sedation and subsequent amnesia during and after the procedure. In patients who have recently eaten, or who have significant gastro-oesophageal reflux, it may be preferable to undertake an RSI and intubation so that the airway is protected. If the patient has acute cardiogenic pulmonary oedema, or is shocked, follow the principles described in the preceding sections.

Sepsis

Patients who have severe sepsis or septic shock may exhibit respiratory distress because of their primary pathology and/or because of the compensatory increase in ventilation that accompanies a severe metabolic acidosis. Indications for intubation remain as for all other conditions, but the patient will be in a precarious balance of high minute ventilation, marked reduction in vascular tone, and a variable cardiac output that is dependent on an adequate intravascular volume and heart rate.

Induction of anaesthesia, institution of positive pressure ventilation and attempts to deliver a minute ventilation sufficient to compensate for severe metabolic acidosis are likely to precipitate cardiovascular collapse.

Early involvement of the intensive care team is essential: invasive arterial and central venous pressure monitoring, vasopressors and inotropes may all be required before RSI.

Anaphylaxis and angio-oedema

Anaphylaxis to any allergen may lead to upper airway obstruction caused by severe oedema. Generally, this initially affects the eyelids, face and lips and makes intubation very difficult.

Early use of adrenaline frequently prevents progression of this condition, but if the patient continues to deteriorate a judgement may have to be made by a senior practitioner to proceed with intubation.

Laryngeal and pharyngeal oedema develop more slowly, but may make it difficult to see the larynx and necessitate intubation with a smaller tracheal tube. Tissues are swollen and friable, so that minor trauma may increase the swelling: gentle use of instruments is essential. These patients have many characteristics that lead to the 'can't intubate, can't ventilate' situation and a clear 'plan B' with all appropriate back-up devices and personnel must be immediately available. Even if the airway is controlled, there may be marked bronchospasm and treatment will be similar to that for severe asthma.

Even though facial swelling may quickly resolve, do not remove the tracheal tube until an audible inspiratory leak at low pressure is evident when the cuff is deflated: by this stage the patient will be in an intensive care unit.

Summary

- There are many cardiorespiratory emergencies requiring urgent induction of anaesthesia and intubation.
- A reduced reservoir of oxygen and impaired cardiovascular reserve amplify the side effects of anaesthetic and sedative drugs.
- Intensive care specialists must be involved at an early stage and, whenever possible, before intubation.
- The dose of induction drugs must be modified carefully to reflect the patient's physiological state: vasoactive drugs will probably be required.
- Conversion from spontaneous to positive pressure ventilation may cause cardiovascular decompensation.

Further reading

1 British Thoracic Society and Scottish Intercollegiate Guidelines Network (2008) *British Guideline on the Management of Asthma. A National Clinical Guideline.* London: British Thoracic Society and Scottish Intercollegiate Guidelines Network. Available at: www.sign.ac.uk/pdf/sign101.pdf

2 National Institute for Health and Clinical Excellence (2004) *Clinical Guideline 12. Chronic Obstructive Pulmonary Disease. Management of Chronic Obstructive Pulmonary Disease in Adults in Primary and Secondary Care.* London: National Institute for Health and Clinical Excellence. Available at: www.nice.org.uk/pdf/ CG012_niceguideline.pdf

3 McLean-Tooke, A. P. C., Bethune, C. A., Fay, A. C. & Spickett, G. P. (2003) Adrenaline in the treatment of anaphylaxis: what is the evidence? *BMJ*; **327**: 1332–5.

4 Resuscitation Council (UK) (2008) Emergency treatment of anaphylactic reactions. London: Resuscitation Council (UK). See: www.resus.org.uk/ pages/reaction.pdf

NON-TRAUMATIC COMA AND SEIZURES
Objectives

The objectives of this section are to:

- understand the immediate risks to the comatose or convulsing patient
- understand the principles of immediate airway management in these patients
- be familiar with the modifications to advanced airway techniques needed in the special circumstances of non-traumatic coma and seizures
- understand what these modifications mean, in practical terms, for the emergency airway practitioner
- be aware of the pitfalls frequently encountered in these patients.

Introduction

Coma is defined as a state of unconsciousness with no reaction to external or internal stimuli, with preservation of some reflex activity. It can be divided into coma of traumatic and non-traumatic origin. The emergency airway management of patients with traumatic coma is described earlier in this chapter in Trauma and raised intracranial pressure. A GCS of eight or less indicates that the patient is in coma; this section focuses on the emergency airway management of patients with non-traumatic coma and seizures.

A general discussion of the diagnosis and treatment of non-traumatic coma and seizures is beyond the scope of this manual, but as an aide memoire some of the common causes of non-traumatic coma are listed in Box 11.2, using the mnemonic COMA. There is often a combination of causes: a patient with alcohol intoxication who has fallen may also have an extradural haematoma.

Box 11.2 Causes of non-traumatic coma (mnemonic: COMA)

Cerebral
- Tumour
- Infection: meningitis, encephalitis, cerebral abscess
- Cerebral haemorrhage: extra/subdural, intracerebral, subarachnoid
- Cerebral/cerebellar ischaemia, infarction
- Post-ictal
- Hydrocephalus

Overdose
- Alcohol, and alcohol withdrawal
- Drugs: opioids, sedatives, hypnotics, salicylates

Metabolic/Endocrine
- Hypoglycaemia or hyperglycaemia
- Electrolyte disturbances: sodium, calcium and magnesium
- Organ failure: renal, hepatic, pulmonary, cardiac
- Diabetic emergencies, thyroid dysfunction, pituitary failure
- Hypothermia

Airway/Asphyxia
- Hypoxaemia
- Hypercarbia

Risks to the comatose or convulsing patient

Comatose patients have depressed neuronal activity within the central nervous system. Neuronal centres responsible for the control of respiratory function, vasomotor tone and protective laryngeal reflexes are attenuated to varying degrees, depending on the cause of the coma. It is, therefore, not surprising that the most significant risks faced by these patients are hypoxaemia, hypercarbia, cardiac dysrhythmias, aspiration of gastric contents, low cardiac output and seizures. Patients undergoing prolonged and uncontrolled grand mal seizures also face the added risks of rhabdomyolysis, hyperthermia and further brain injury secondary to more severe hypoxaemia and central metabolic acidosis from the hypercatabolic state caused by the seizures.

Immediate treatment principles

In the first instance, efforts are directed at creating and maintaining a patent airway to enable delivery of a high concentration of inspired oxygen. For some comatose patients, simple airway manoeuvres (chin lift or jaw thrust), basic adjuncts (oropharyngeal and/or nasopharyngeal airways), high-flow oxygen via a facemask with reservoir bag, and close observation may be all that is necessary. Examples of this scenario include the hypoglycaemic patient before treatment, or coma secondary to opioid overdose before naloxone has been given. In an epileptic patient with a self-limiting grand mal seizure, airway protection from aspiration is rarely required because the unco-ordinated motor activity precludes co-ordinated expulsion of gastric contents, and protective laryngeal reflexes return early during the recovery phase. Positioning the patient on their side on a tipping trolley, suctioning secretions and blood, the application of a jaw thrust or insertion of a nasopharyngeal airway to relieve obstruction by the tongue are usually all that is necessary.

Where hypoventilation occurs in a patient with non-traumatic coma, ventilation using a bag-mask device may be necessary to maintain oxygenation and prevent hypercarbia, before securing a definitive airway. Whether the person performing this task possesses the skills necessary to secure a definitive airway or not, it will also effectively begin the process of pre-oxygenation before RSI and intubation, maximizing the patient's chances of a good outcome.

During initial airway management, thought should be given to identifying the underlying cause of the coma. At best it may be reversible, or it may be possible to improve the level of consciousness, thereby avoiding the need to intubate. Furthermore, knowledge of the underlying diagnosis may influence the technique used for securing the airway.

Try to obtain as much history about the patient as is feasible given the clinical circumstances.

- Sudden collapse with coma implies a neurovascular cause (ischaemic or haemorrhagic stroke, subarachnoid haemorrhage) or cardiac arrhythmia.
- Gradual deterioration (minutes to a few hours) into coma is associated more frequently with metabolic causes and drug intoxication.
- Evidence of drug overdose is often found at the scene. Seek information from pre-hospital personnel wherever possible.
- Deterioration into coma over a longer period is more usually associated with infection and organ failure (hepatic, respiratory, renal or endocrine).

The urgency of the situation may preclude a full physical examination and a rapid initial assessment may be all that can be achieved before securing a definitive airway. In these circumstances the full general examination is deferred until the airway is secured.

Consider raised ICP in any patient who has reduced consciousness. Further confirmatory signs of an increased ICP may also be apparent in the rapid initial assessment of the comatose or seizing patient (Box 11.3). In these circumstances techniques to reduce the pressor response to laryngoscopy and intubation will form part of the RSI.

Box 11.3 Signs of raised intracranial pressure

- Reduced consciousness
- Irregular or slow respiratory pattern
- Hypertension and bradycardia
- Extensor posturing
- Papilloedema
- Pupillary signs

Measure the capillary or venous glucose, record the patient's temperature, and take an arterial blood sample if time permits. This frequently provides information that will inform the immediate management plan and act as a baseline against which further results can be compared.

Indications for intubation in the non-traumatic coma or convulsing patient

Determining when to proceed from supportive airway measures to intubation is one of the key challenges clinicians face when managing patients in coma of non-traumatic origin, or those who are seizing. As a general rule the decision to intubate is made when the risks of not intervening outweigh the risks of doing so. Clinical experience aids the decision-making process. Box 11.4 lists the absolute and relative indications for securing a definitive airway in these patients.

There is no clear guideline that defines specifically the duration of generalized seizure activity before there is a need to intubate the patient. In UK practice, most experienced clinicians would consider tracheal intubation in those patients with seizures lasting more than 15 minutes following hospital arrival, and refractory to first-line anticonvulsant therapy (benzodiazepines). In patients with an established diagnosis of epilepsy, second-line anticonvulsant therapy is usually commenced (e.g. phenytoin) before intubation. When there is no previous history of seizures the need for CT scanning of the head usually brings forward the decision to intubate.

The technique of tracheal intubation
The comatose patient

Although it may be physically possible to intubate the comatose patient without using drugs, this is seldom advisable. Intubating conditions will be far from ideal, and apart from the risk of trauma and laryngospasm, autonomic reflex

---

Box 11.4 Indications for tracheal intubation in non-traumatic coma and seizures

Failure to maintain a patent airway:
- obstruction despite the use of basic manoeuvres and adjuncts
- lack of protective laryngeal reflexes
- seizures refractory to treatment, compromising the airway.

Failure of ventilation:
- apnoea
- hypoxaemia ($SpO_2 < 92\%$, $PaO_2 < 9$ kPa) on supplemental oxygen (60%)
- hypercarbia ($PaCO_2 > 6.5$ kPa).

Prolonged seizure activity:
- includes generalized status epilepticus, refractory to anticonvulsant treatment.

To facilitate treatment of the underlying condition:
- intracranial haemorrhage with raised ICP
- tricyclic antidepressant overdose with a metabolic acidosis and/or GCS < 9
- high-risk patients who require CT scanning
- patients who require transportation.

---

activity will cause an increase in blood pressure and ICP. Either or both of these may worsen the underlying cause of coma or precipitate further complications, for example:

- hypertension may cause further bleeding after an intracerebral haemorrhage
- a rise in ICP may cause coning.

Rapid sequence induction is, therefore, the technique of choice for securing the airway in this group of patients with the following considerations.

Pre-oxygenation Pre-existing hypoxaemia ($PaO_2 < 8$ kPa, 60 mmHg) will cause an increase in cerebral blood flow and ICP, and may also be contributing to the decreased level of consciousness. If the patient's spontaneous ventilatory efforts are severely impaired, assisted ventilation will be required to improve the effectiveness of pre-oxygenation. Use small tidal volumes and low inflation pressures to avoid gastric distension and an increased risk of regurgitation.

Cricoid pressure Application of cricoid pressure is indicated because there may not have been time for the stomach to empty before the onset of coma, and many causes of coma delay gastric emptying, e.g. opioids, salicylate poisoning, hypoxaemia, hyperglycaemia, hypothermia, increased ICP.

Drugs for induction of anaesthesia Thiopental sodium, etomidate and propofol are suitable for use in most comatose patients. A reduced dose will be required, particularly when coma is drug induced, or in the presence of hypovolaemia.

Neuromuscular blocking drugs Suxamethonium remains the drug of choice in almost all cases. The use of suxamethonium has been questioned when the ICP is known to be high, but when given with an anaesthetic induction drug, suxamethonium causes a negligible increase in ICP.

Adjuvant treatment Intravenous opioids given before the induction of anaesthesia will attenuate the autonomic reflexes that cause an increase in blood pressure and ICP. The opioids most commonly used are fentanyl and alfentanil, given one to three minutes before laryngoscopy (see Chapter 8).

The convulsing patient

The motor manifestations of seizures can be stopped and muscle relaxation achieved to facilitate tracheal intubation by giving neuromuscular blocking drugs alone. This is totally inappropriate as neuronal seizure activity will continue and the patient will suffer the adverse consequences associated with the cardiovascular response to intubation. Furthermore, should seizures stop, either spontaneously or as a result of treatment given, there is a risk of the patient being paralysed and aware. Consequently, both an intravenous induction drug and a neuromuscular blocking drug must be given. It is also important to consider that patients who are fitting may have vomited or bitten their lips or tongue: there may be vomit or blood in the airway that will make intubation more difficult. A wide-bore rigid sucker (e.g. Yankauer type) must always be immediately available. The technique of tracheal intubation follows that described in Chapter 7, with the following additional considerations.

Pre-oxygenation This may be difficult to achieve because of unco-ordinated respiratory effort and myoclonus of the upper airway, oropharynx and muscles of mastication. An attempt should be made, even if it is only possible to apply high-flow oxygen to the patient's mouth and nose. Because of this potential difficulty, time to desaturation during the initial intubation attempt may be short.

Drugs for the induction of anaesthesia Thiopental sodium has profound anticonvulsant activity and will terminate most seizures at the dose used to induce unconsciousness. It also causes marked myocardial depression, and therefore a reduced dose may be required in some circumstances. Etomidate may raise the seizure threshold in grand mal seizures, but lowers the threshold in focal seizures. However, patients with focal seizures rarely require emergency airway management. Although propofol may cause myoclonic activity, it has anticonvulsant properties and is an acceptable alternative.

Adjuvant treatment The same considerations apply as for the comatose patient.

Pitfalls

1 Failure to recognize and treat hypoglycaemia and opioid overdose.

2 Failure to recognize the importance of the anticipated clinical course. This is particularly true in cases of deliberate poisoning with tricyclic antidepressants, anticonvulsants and antiarrhythmics. By considering the pharmacodynamic and pharmacokinetic profiles of the ingested substance, and an approximate time of ingestion, it is possible to predict with reasonable certainty when the clinical state of the patient is likely to worsen. Early intervention, including intubation and ventilation with intensive care support, when the patient is more tolerant of the cardiovascular side effects of the drugs used, is preferable to acting later in an increasingly unstable patient.

3 The paralysed patient can still be fitting, and will therefore require effective sedation (e.g. midazolam) along with anticonvulsants. Continuous bedside EEG enables monitoring of seizure activity and response to treatment. In most cases it will be necessary to allow motor recovery to occur to assess the response to anticonvulsant treatment. In the sedated, paralysed patient, bursts of hypertension, tachycardia and pupillary dilatation are suggestive of seizure activity.

4 New prolonged seizure activity usually represents a significant change in seizure behaviour for the patient. Look for an underlying cause (e.g. metabolic, infective, cerebrovascular event).

Summary

- Patients who are in coma of a non-traumatic origin, or fitting, often present specific problems to the airway practitioner.
- The method for securing a definitive airway in these patients is modified according to the particular circumstances of each case.
- Early recognition of the high risk of these patients, awareness of the potential pitfalls and a team-based approach will maximize the chances of obtaining a good patient outcome.

Further reading

1 Grange, C. & Watson, D. (1997) Coma: initial assessment and management. In: *Cambridge Textbook of Emergency Medicine*, eds. Skinner, D., Swain, A., Peyton, R. & Robertson, C. Cambridge: Cambridge University Press.

2 Jordan, K. G. (1999) Convulsive and nonconvulsive status epilepticus in the intensive care unit and emergency department. In: *Critical Care Neurology (Blue Book of Practical Neurology – 22)*, eds. Miller, D. H. & Raps, E. C. Boston: Butterworth-Heinemann.

3 Bradford, J. C. & Kyriakedes, C. G. (1999) Evaluation of the patient with seizures: an evidence based approach. *Emerg Med Clin North Am*; **17**: 203–20.

4 Huff, J. S., Morris, D. L., Kothari, R. U. & Gibbs, M. A. (2001) Emergency Medicine Seizure Study Group. Emergency department management of patients with seizures: a multicenter study. *Acad Emerg Med*; **8**: 622–8.

PRE-HOSPITAL CARE
Objectives
The objectives of this section are to:
- understand the background and principles of pre-hospital RSI and tracheal intubation
- understand the differences between in-hospital and pre-hospital RSI, and the potential problems that are unique to this environment.

Background
The procedure of pre-hospital RSI is carried out to a greater or lesser extent in the majority of European countries. In the UK, it is carried out only by doctors working in pre-hospital care, and relatively infrequently. Worldwide, pre-hospital intubation is carried out in several ways by a variety of practitioners. The procedure is performed with and without drugs. When drugs are used they may consist of a benzodiazepine only or an induction drug with a neuromuscular blocking drug. Practitioners include paramedics, nurses and doctors. Paramedics have markedly different experience and training in different systems. Doctors need to be aware of the possible indications for pre-hospital RSI and the potential hazards of the procedure outside the usual hospital environment. The subject of pre-hospital RSI is not supported by a high-quality evidence base.

Pre-hospital rapid sequence induction in an emergency medical service
Pre-hospital RSI should not be undertaken by individuals working in isolation; it should be part of a well-organized system. A system supporting the procedure needs to provide the following elements:
- a structure to ensure that practitioners are competent to perform the procedure
- control, support and supervision of practitioners
- training and continuing education
- standard guidelines or protocols
- techniques and equipment that bring the procedure as close as possible to standards achieved in hospital (e.g. national standards of anaesthetic monitoring)
- audit and quality assurance programmes.

Indications
The *possible* indications for pre-hospital RSI are essentially the same as for RSI in the emergency department. These are discussed comprehensively in Chapter 5. In every case a rapid but careful on-scene risk/benefit assessment is made, and the potential benefits of pre-hospital RSI are balanced against the risks of the procedure in a given scenario. Examples of factors influencing the decision might include the experience of the practitioner, assistance available, the time to hospital, the effect of basic airway manoeuvres, expected clinical course or anticipated difficulties with the procedure (e.g. an anticipated difficult intubation).

While some situations will require little consideration (e.g. where gross hypoxaemia exists despite basic airway manoeuvres, and airway reflexes prevent non-drug assisted intubation), in others the potential benefit may be less clear.

Principles

1 Patients in near or actual cardiorespiratory arrest, where airway reflexes are lost, may be intubated without drugs, following simple airway manoeuvres and bag-mask ventilation.

2 The only absolute indication for pre-hospital RSI is total failure to establish a patent airway by any other means, in a patient who requires drug administration to counter airway reflexes. This is an extremely rare event.

3 In all other cases, the potential benefits of RSI must be weighed against the potential risks. Pre-hospital practitioners work in a highly exposed situation, and RSI requires significant time, which may exceed the journey time to the nearest hospital.

4 In general, if the airway is adequate, pre-hospital RSI is not required. Exceptions might be a prolonged transport time, or where the anticipated clinical course is one of rapid deterioration (e.g. airway burns).

Technique

Key considerations in the technique of pre-hospital RSI
- Safety
- Patient access
- Patient positioning
- Environment
- Equipment
- Assistance

Safety

As in all pre-hospital care, safety is of paramount importance. Safety considerations extend to the practitioner, colleagues on scene and the patient(s). On no account should RSI be undertaken in an area that is, or may become, unsafe. This may require the patient to be moved before RSI.

Patient access

Good patient access is essential, particularly if difficulties are encountered. It is helpful to consider what will happen if a surgical airway is required. In general, it is not appropriate to attempt intubation before extrication (e.g. from a crashed vehicle) unless all other attempts to maintain the airway have failed: in the vast majority of cases airway intervention should be restricted to simple manoeuvres and provision of oxygen until extrication and full patient access can be achieved. Give drugs to trapped or inaccessible persons only with extreme caution since these may precipitate deterioration in a previously adequate airway, which cannot then be restored. While RSI may be undertaken in an ambulance, there is a risk of compromising both access and positioning because of the relatively cramped conditions. This must be balanced against the weather protection and light that are provided within a vehicle.

Patient positioning

It is difficult to intubate a patient lying on the floor or on their side: in general, the practitioner will have to lie prone. In some circumstances, such as where gross hypoxaemia exists despite basic airway manoeuvres, then there may be little alternative. Where possible, move the patient to a more convenient height, usually on an ambulance trolley. Ensure that all equipment remains readily to hand: if this is laid out on the floor then the patient should be at a height where a kneeling practitioner can comfortably intubate the patient.

Environment

Sunlight will cause the practitioner's pupils to constrict, making subsequent laryngoscopy very difficult: the patient and practitioner should therefore be shaded for the procedure. Conversely, the patient will become very cold in a wet or wintry environment, particularly following intubation and paralysis. Beware of groups of curious bystanders, friends or relations: they can become interfering or hostile, particularly if things do not seem to be going well.

Equipment

Much of the equipment taken for granted in hospitals is either not available or less reliable in the pre-hospital environment. It is essential to ensure that adequate oxygen, suction and monitoring (including end tidal CO_2 measurement) are available, and that everything that might be required (including surgical airway equipment) is available and fully functional. Colourimetric carbon dioxide detectors, which provide visual confirmation of carbon dioxide with the first breath following intubation, are invaluable.

Assistance

Skilled assistance is often less readily available, particularly in pre-hospital systems where RSI is not commonplace. Rapid sequence induction should be undertaken only with trained assistance. Additional people may also be required to provide skills such as manual stabilization of the cervical spine.

Summary
- Pre-hospital RSI should be carried out only in an organized and supportive system.
- Each pre-hospital RSI should be performed only after a risk/benefit assessment.

- The indications for pre-hospital RSI are similar to those in hospital, but their application will depend upon several factors that are specific to each situation. These include the experience of the practitioner, assistance available, the transport time to hospital, the patient's condition and anticipated clinical course.
- The practitioner must be familiar with the unique aspects of pre-hospital care and with RSI before undertaking this procedure.

Further reading

1 Lockey, D. & Porter, K. (2007) Prehospital anaesthesia in the UK: position statement on behalf of the Faculty of Pre-hospital Care. *Emerg Med J*; **24**: 606–7.

12

Non-invasive ventilatory support

Alasdair Gray, Jerry Nolan and Carl Gwinnutt

Objectives

The objectives of this chapter are to understand:

- the mechanisms of action of non-invasive ventilation
- the clinical applications for non-invasive ventilation in the acute setting
- the role of continuous positive airway pressure (CPAP) versus bi-level positive airway pressure (BiPAP)
- the limitations and complications of non-invasive ventilation (NIV)
- the practical application of NIV.

Introduction

NIV is the provision of ventilatory support through the patient's upper airway using a mask or similar device. Non-invasive application of CPAP does not, strictly speaking, constitute ventilatory support but in this chapter it is included under the generic term NIV. Use of NIV may avoid the need for intubation and invasive ventilation; it is also used to supplement medical therapy. There is good evidence supporting its use in patients with chronic obstructive pulmonary disease (COPD) with moderate dyspnoea and hypercapnia, and in acute cardiogenic pulmonary oedema. Non-invasive ventilation may be used in patients who are not suitable for intubation, and considered for patients with hypoxaemic respiratory failure such as asthma or community acquired pneumonia.

Modes of non-invasive ventilation

There are several different terms describing the modes of non-invasive ventilation – this terminology is confusing. Based on the level of respiratory support, the modes include:

- CMV, which requires no patient effort
- assisted spontaneous breathing or pressure support, which increases ventilation support but relies on the patient's spontaneous respiratory effort
- CPAP, during which a constant positive pressure is applied throughout the respiratory cycle.

Combinations of these modes are available. A combination of pressure support and CPAP is known as bi-level pressure support or BiPAP. This chapter

Emergency Airway Management, eds. Jonathan Benger, Jerry Nolan and Mike Clancy.
Published by Cambridge University Press. © College of Emergency Medicine, London 2009.

focuses on CPAP and BiPAP, because these are the modes used most commonly outside intensive care.

Mechanisms of action
Continuous positive airway pressure
Continuous positive airway pressure is typically used to correct hypoxaemia in type 1 respiratory failure ($PaO_2 < 8$ kPa with a normal or low $PaCO_2$). It has several mechanisms of action.

- Increase in functional residual capacity (FRC) – the volume of gas remaining in the lungs at the end of a normal expiration. A low FRC causes atelectasis and lung collapse, leading to ventilation/perfusion (V/Q) mismatch and reduced pulmonary compliance with increased airway resistance. This increases the work of breathing. Restoration of the FRC towards normal improves oxygenation and reduces the work of breathing.

- Reopening closed or under ventilated alveoli (recruitment). This occurs as part of the general improvement in FRC and reduces intrapulmonary shunting (perfusion of unventilated alveoli), thereby improving oxygenation.

- Reduction in left ventricular transmural pressure. This is of value in left ventricular failure, and may be the main mechanism by which CPAP improves oxygenation in acute cardiogenic pulmonary oedema. It also reduces afterload and preload, to which the failing heart is sensitive. Continuous positive airway pressure does not necessarily drive pulmonary oedema fluid back into the circulation, and total lung water may not change despite clinical improvement.

- Reducing threshold work. In patients with auto-PEEP (intrinsic positive end expiratory pressure) or dynamic hyperinflation, the inspiratory muscles have to work to drop the alveolar pressure from its positive, end-expiratory value to less than the upper airway pressure (normally zero) before inspiratory gas flow occurs. This is termed threshold work, and may be significant. By increasing the airway pressure, CPAP reduces the work required to initiate inspiratory flow. This may reduce respiratory rate and $PaCO_2$, and is the reason that CPAP is sometimes considered to provide ventilatory support as well as correction of hypoxaemia.

- Airway splinting. Continuous positive airway pressure is a specific treatment for obstructive sleep apnoea, and is often of value in patients with temporary airway problems.

- Delivery of high FiO_2. Efficient CPAP systems deliver oxygen at flows that exceed the patient's peak inspiratory flow, without rebreathing; thus the selected inspired oxygen concentration (up to 100%) is delivered reliably.

Bi-level positive airway pressure
Bi-level positive airway pressure is a combination of CPAP with pressure support. Two pressure settings are selected: a higher, inspiratory positive airway pressure (IPAP), and a lower, expiratory positive airway pressure (EPAP). The difference between them generates a tidal volume (ventilation). Expiratory positive airway

pressure is effectively CPAP – it recruits under ventilated alveoli and increases FRC (improving oxygenation), and reduces threshold work in the presence of auto-PEEP (see above). When the patient is breathing spontaneously, the patient's respiratory effort triggers both the inspiratory and expiratory phase of the respiratory cycle. In this mode, if the patient develops apnoea, no respiratory assistance will occur; however, many BiPAP machines incorporate a back-up rate of six to eight breaths per minute. In timed mode, mandatory breaths are delivered, although patient triggering is also possible. Use of BiPAP decreases respiratory rate and work of breathing, and improves alveolar ventilation.

Clinical uses

In the acute setting, the two principal indications for NIV are acute exacerbations of COPD and acute cardiogenic pulmonary oedema. Other indications include chest wall deformity and neuromuscular disease, decompensated sleep apnoea, chest trauma, pneumonia and to assist weaning in the intensive care unit.

Chronic obstructive pulmonary disease

Consider using BiPAP in patients with an acute exacerbation of COPD, an acute respiratory acidosis (pH < 7.35; $H^+ > 45$ nmol l^{-1}), and who remain acidotic despite maximal medical treatment on controlled oxygen therapy. Give oxygen to maintain the oxygen saturation of arterial blood between 87% and 92%; an excessive inspired oxygen concentration may increase CO_2 retention. In approximately 50% of patients who are initially acidotic on arrival in the emergency department, blood gas values will be returned to baseline in response to this treatment. Typical BiPAP settings are described below.

Despite some case series documenting beneficial effects of CPAP in the treatment of acute exacerbations of COPD, it is conventional practice to use BiPAP in this situation.

Cardiogenic pulmonary oedema

Continuous positive airway pressure is widely used for the treatment of patients presenting with acute cardiogenic pulmonary oedema. It improves physiology by the mechanisms outlined above. Rates of intubation, but not mortality, are reduced. Consider the use of BiPAP in patients with acute cardiogenic pulmonary oedema who fail to improve with CPAP, particularly if they are hypercapnic. Some BiPAP machines will not deliver oxygen at a concentration high enough to maintain adequate oxygenation of arterial blood.

Patient suitability

Several factors predict success in patients with acute respiratory failure who require non-invasive ventilatory support. These include less severe physiological derangement and less pre-existing co-morbidity; an improvement in pH, $PaCO_2$ and respiratory rate after one hour of NIV; and a high-quality patient–machine interface. Some patients are unable to tolerate tight-fitting facemasks – nasal masks are available, but these are generally less efficient (the patient must be able to keep their mouth closed) and are not commonly used in the acute setting. Non-invasive ventilation helmets have recently become available, and may be better tolerated. Some patients have difficulty synchronizing their breathing with the NIV system. Facial anatomy influences the success of NIV: edentulous patients may have particular difficulties with a facemask.

Contraindications

The most important contraindication to the use of NIV is the need for immediate tracheal intubation and conventional ventilation. Many of the factors previously considered to be contraindications are relative – with experience, the boundaries for the use of NIV are expanding, e.g. after application of BiPAP the obtunded patient with an acute exacerbation of COPD may quickly become more conscious as the $PaCO_2$ decreases. Many contraindications are negated if tracheal intubation is considered inappropriate and NIV is to be used as the 'ceiling' of treatment. Other important contraindications to NIV include:

- facial trauma or burns
- fixed obstruction of the upper airway
- vomiting.

   Relative contraindications include:

- recent facial, upper airway, or upper gastro-intestinal tract surgery
- inability to protect the airway
- haemodynamic instability
- severe co-morbidity
- impaired consciousness
- confusion or agitation
- bowel obstruction
- copious respiratory secretions
- undrained pneumothorax.

   Non-invasive ventilation may be used in these circumstances, particularly if tracheal intubation is not deemed appropriate.

Complications

If patients are selected correctly, the majority of complications are relatively minor. Potential complications of NIV include:

- hypotension: an increase in intrathoracic pressure reduces right ventricular end diastolic volume and can cause hypotension, particularly if there is hypovolaemia
- barotrauma: over inflation and gas trapping are possible, although pneumothorax is rare
- discomfort: patients frequently find the facemask uncomfortable and claustrophobic
- gastric distension: although NIV can cause gastric inflation, prophylactic placement of a nasogastric tube is not required in every patient

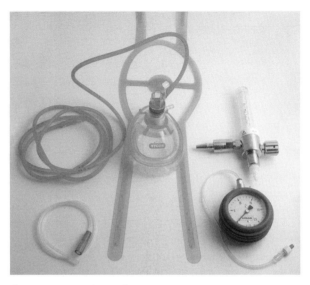

Figure 12.1 A Boussignac valve.

- pulmonary aspiration: vomiting or regurgitation into a tight-fitting facemask may cause massive aspiration
- pressure necrosis: this may be prevented by the use of a hydrocolloid or similar dressing placed over vulnerable areas such as the bridge of the nose. This problem is much less common with modern NIV masks.

Environment

Patients treated with NIV should be managed in an environment with suitable monitoring, including continuous pulse oximetry, access to equipment for blood gas analysis and immediate availability of resuscitation equipment. Staff should be fully trained in the use of NIV. Personnel skilled in tracheal intubation should be available with minimal delay.

Equipment

Figure 12.1 shows a simple CPAP valve that is easy to use and can deliver almost 100% oxygen.

Figure 12.2 shows a typical portable non-invasive ventilator that is able to provide both CPAP and BiPAP. These ventilators were designed initially for home ventilation: they are simple to use and usually portable. However, because air is entrained with high-flow oxygen in an open circuit, it is not possible to measure FiO_2 or deliver an FiO_2 of greater than 50–60%.

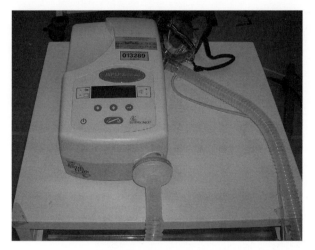

Figure 12.2 Respironics Synchrony non-invasive ventilator.

A more sophisticated ventilator is shown in Figure 12.3. This will provide CPAP and BiPAP with an FiO_2 of up to 100%. This machine has significant monitoring capabilities, but it is more complicated to use, not portable and significantly more expensive than alternatives.

Several patient–machine interfaces are available, including nasal masks, face-masks and helmets. The most widely used interface in an emergency setting is the facemask. The mask must be sized and fitted correctly, and not applied too tightly. Most modern NIV machines and masks are designed to allow some leakage around the mask to improve patient triggering and tolerance. The correct position of the mask is illustrated in Figure 12.4.

Procedure

- With the patient sitting, turn on the NIV system and gas flow, set the desired oxygen concentration, select the correct size of facemask and apply it to the patient's face. Patient acceptance may be facilitated if the mask is applied manually for the first few minutes.
- Once the patient is comfortable with the system, apply the straps to produce a snug, but not excessively tight, fit.
- When using CPAP, start with a pressure of 5–10 cmH$_2$O and titrate up to 15 cmH$_2$0 depending on the patient's oxygen saturation, respiratory rate and the degree of mask leak.
- When using BiPAP, typical initial ventilator settings are EPAP 3–5 cmH$_2$O and IPAP 12–15 cmH$_2$O, which can be increased as tolerated up to 20 cmH$_2$O.

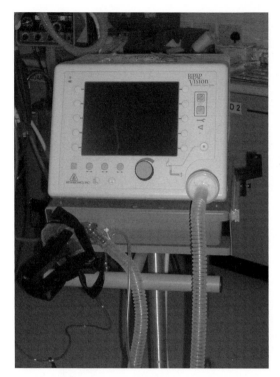

Figure 12.3 Respironics Vision non-invasive ventilator.

- Observe the patient closely and assess: chest wall movement, co-ordination of respiratory effort with the ventilator, accessory muscle recruitment, respiratory rate, heart rate, patient comfort and mental state.
- Monitor the oxygen saturation continuously and measure the arterial blood gas values after 30 minutes to 1 hour. The frequency of subsequent arterial blood gas analysis will depend on the patient's response to treatment.
- If the patient has COPD, titrate the FiO_2 to an oxygen saturation of 88–92%.

Failure of non-invasive ventilatory support

If CPAP fails to improve the patient's oxygenation and respiratory rate, consider the need for tracheal intubation to enable application of higher positive end expiratory pressure (PEEP) and other modes of ventilation. If CPAP has produced adequate oxygenation but the patient is tiring and the $PaCO_2$ is rising,

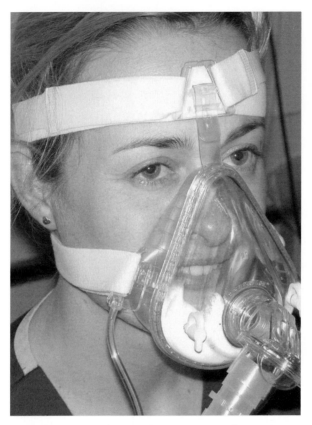

Figure 12.4 Correct mask position for non-invasive ventilatory support.

consider the use of non-invasive BiPAP or tracheal intubation. A deteriorating $PaCO_2$, pH, respiratory rate or conscious level, despite the use of BiPAP, will necessitate an alternative treatment strategy. This might include BiPAP in a timed (mandatory) mode or, if appropriate, tracheal intubation.

Summary
- Consider BiPAP for patients with acute exacerbations of COPD, and CPAP for those with acute cardiogenic pulmonary oedema.
- Do not use NIV if there is an indication for immediate tracheal intubation, and intubation is appropriate.

Further reading

1 Mehta, S. & Hill, N. (2001) Noninvasive ventilation. *Am J Respir Crit Care Med*; **163**: 540–77.
2 British Thoracic Society Standards of Care Committee (2002) BTS guideline: non-invasive ventilation in acute respiratory failure. *Thorax*; **57**: 192–211.
3 Agarwal, R., Aggarwal, A.N., Gupta, D. & Jindal, S.J. (2005) Non-invasive ventilation in acute cardiogenic pulmonary oedema. *Postgrad Med J*; **81**: 637–43.

Acknowledgement

Steve Crane supplied Figures 12.1, 12.2 and 12.3.

The interface between departments and hospitals

Jerry Nolan, Mike Clancy and Jonathan Benger

Objective

The objective of this chapter is to:

• consider the interface between the emergency department and other hospital departments in relation to advanced airway management.

Introduction

A successful programme for advanced airway management outside the operating theatre is dependent on collaboration between several hospital departments. Collaboration is required to establish an effective airway management training programme, to undertake advanced airway management appropriately and safely, to enhance the transfer of patient care from the emergency department to the receiving team and to enable continued practice in airway management. The interface between the emergency department, the intensive care unit (ICU) and the anaesthesia department is particularly important.

Interface with the intensive care unit

Data provided by the Intensive Care National Audit and Research Centre (ICNARC) indicate that 26% of admissions to the ICU come through the emergency department. Just over three quarters of these are admitted directly from the emergency department. Early referral of critically ill patients to the intensive care team is vitally important. Whenever possible intensivists should be involved in the decision to anaesthetize and intubate a patient: they are likely to be responsible for taking on the patient's subsequent care.

The intubation decision

The decision to admit a patient to the ICU will depend on their severity of illness, their pre-existing functional capacity and physiological reserve, and the reversibility of the acute illness. In some cases, in particular those with severe, progressive, chronic disease, intubation will be inappropriate because of the limited chance of long-term survival. Some patients may have indicated before their acute deterioration that they would not wish to be intubated or placed on ventilatory support. Emergency physicians and intensivists will gain the relevant information to assist decision-making from the patient, relatives, the general

Emergency Airway Management, eds. Jonathan Benger, Jerry Nolan and Mike Clancy.
Published by Cambridge University Press. © College of Emergency Medicine, London 2009.

practitioner and from medical records. If in doubt about the patient's chances of long-term survival, and if the patient's wishes are unknown, intubation and other life-sustaining interventions should be undertaken. Some patients will be better treated with non-invasive respiratory support: early involvement of intensivists will enable these decisions to be made before the patient deteriorates to the point at which tracheal intubation becomes the only option.

Tracheal intubation
Either team can undertake advanced airway management, but it is sensible to maximize the educational opportunity and enable a practitioner in training to undertake the rapid sequence induction and intubation in the presence of an experienced individual. Induction of anaesthesia in the critically ill is hazardous and all healthcare staff must work together to ensure optimal fluid resuscitation and use of inotropic and other drugs.

Transfer
Early discussion with the intensive care team is essential, as this will enable a management plan to be established. This might include transfer to the CT scanner or operating theatre before admission to the ICU. Patients may need to be transferred to another hospital for clinical reasons: e.g. referral to neurosurgical, burns or cardiothoracic units. There is a well-recognized shortage of intensive care beds in the UK and, very occasionally, this will force transfer of the intubated patient to another hospital for a non-clinical reason. Most intensive care networks now operate a policy whereby a more stable, existing ICU patient would be transferred, thus making a bed available for the less stable emergency department patient. Even if a bed can be made available in the same hospital, it is not uncommon for critically ill intubated patients to remain for several hours in the resuscitation room while another patient is transferred from the ICU to the ward or to another ICU. On these occasions, emergency physicians and intensive care staff will be working together to treat the patient optimally before arrival in the ICU.

Combined audit and mortality and morbidity meetings involving intensive care and emergency medicine staff are valuable for improving patient care, and for enhancing the collaboration between departments. This feedback on outcomes is the best way for doctors and nurses of all disciplines to learn from their actions.

In the future, collaboration between emergency physicians and intensivists may be extended to include outreach care and medical emergency teams (METs). Effective airway management is an essential skill for any MET, and an appropriately skilled emergency physician could provide this.

Interface with the department of anaesthesia
In the UK, anaesthetists have traditionally undertaken advanced airway management in the emergency department. It is now increasingly common for emergency physicians and anaesthetists to work together to induce anaesthesia and secure

the airway of critically ill patients. Advanced airway management skills are best gained by undertaking a period as a trainee in anaesthesia. Following the implementation of Modernising Medical Careers (MMC), emergency physicians and other trainees opting for acute care common stem (ACCS) rotations gain a total of two years' experience in emergency medicine, anaesthesia, critical care and acute medicine.

Maintenance of advanced airway management skills will require practice. In a busy emergency department this may be achieved within the resuscitation room, but many individuals are unlikely to maintain their skills without visiting the operating theatre for additional practice. Strong liaison between emergency departments and anaesthesia departments will help emergency physicians to maintain airway skills. Training on simulators will also help to maintain skills, and provides another opportunity for anaesthetists and emergency physicians to practice as a team.

Interface with the radiology department

Many critically ill patients will require urgent CT scans (e.g. major trauma, neurological emergencies), and many of these will require rapid sequence induction and intubation to ensure that their airway and ventilation is optimized during the scan. Close liaison with the radiology department will help to minimize the time that the critically ill intubated patient is kept waiting for a scan. Careful planning will also minimize the time that the radiology team is kept waiting for the emergency patient, and will enable other patients to have access to the scanner until the moment the intubated patient is ready. Emergency and intensive care teams should work together to make sure that the CT scan room is properly equipped for the mechanically ventilated patient. This includes appropriate oxygen outlets for the ventilator, power supplies and stands for infusion pumps, and a designated location for the patient monitor so that it remains visible from the control room.

Interface with the ear, nose and throat department

Some patients with severe airway problems may need urgent assessment by an experienced ear, nose and throat (ENT) surgeon. These specialists are particularly adept at nasendoscopy and assessment of the airway. This may be very valuable for assessing patients who are thought to have upper airway obstruction. Direct visualization of the airway will help emergency physicians and anaesthetists to establish a management plan. In some cases, the results of nasendoscopy will enable the patient to be admitted safely to the ICU for close observation, while in others it may reveal a precarious airway and the need for immediate awake fibreoptic intubation.

Interface with the paediatric department

The resuscitation of critically ill children is particularly challenging. Rapid sequence induction of anaesthesia and intubation should be undertaken only by individuals experienced with this procedure in children. Paediatricians will be involved in the resuscitation of any child, and close collaboration between paediatricians, emergency physicians and the intensive care team is essential to enable advanced airway management to be undertaken safely. Training together on courses such as the Advanced Paediatric Life Support (APLS) course will help these specialists work together as a cohesive team. The regionalization of paediatric intensive care services now means that in many cases critically ill children will be transferred to a paediatric intensive care unit (PICU) in another hospital. Most of these units will deploy a retrieval team to collect the patient from the referring hospital. Close collaboration with the regional PICU and the implementation of prearranged protocols will ensure that this transfer is as smooth as possible.

The interface with other hospitals

Some critically ill patients will require transfer to another hospital for further treatment. This may be because of a lack of intensive care beds locally, or because of the need for specialized treatment such as that provided by regional neurosurgical, burns or cardiothoracic units. The anaesthetized intubated patient must be accompanied by someone experienced in advanced airway management (see Chapter 10). Regional units will often have treatment protocols, which they encourage clinicians to follow. Clinicians in the emergency department must liaise closely with staff at the receiving hospital to ensure that an appropriate bed is available.

Summary

- Training in emergency airway management, and putting these acquired skills into practice in the resuscitation room, requires close collaboration between several hospital departments.
- The specialists involved most closely with emergency physicians in the provision of airway management are those from the ICU.

Further reading

1 Simpson, H.K., Clancy, M., Goldfrad, C. & Rowan, K. (2005) Admissions to intensive care units from emergency departments: a descriptive study. *Emerg Med J*; **22**: 423–8.

14

Audit and skills maintenance

Colin Graham

Objectives

The objectives of this chapter are to:
- understand the need for personal and departmental audit of emergency airway interventions
- review skills maintenance requirements for the emergency airway practitioner.

Introduction

Advanced airway skills form the cornerstone of resuscitation. Experience in anaesthesia, intensive care and emergency medicine is invaluable when obtaining these skills; however, it is also necessary to continually audit individual and departmental performance. In this way, any personal or institutional problems can be identified and resolved at an early stage.

Principles of clinical audit

Clinical audit is the monitoring of specific interventions against agreed standards of care. Deviations from the agreed standards can be identified and investigated to determine the cause of problems, which enables solutions to be implemented.

Clinical audit can also be used to drive a quality improvement process for a department or hospital. The structure, process and outcome of emergency airway care can all be audited (Box 14.1).

Box 14.1 Audit of emergency airway care

Structure: audit of availability of specific equipment, e.g. capnography
Process: audit of intubation practice, e.g. personal logbook
Outcome: critical review of cases where more than two attempts are needed to secure the airway

---

Personal audit

Every practitioner should maintain a personal record of emergency airway interventions, which can be presented to a trainer, faculty or college as an indication of experience achieved. This record enables identification of areas of weakness, which can then be addressed. An example of this is given in Box 14.2. Personal records can also form the basis of departmental audit.

Emergency Airway Management, eds. Jonathan Benger, Jerry Nolan and Mike Clancy.
Published by Cambridge University Press. © College of Emergency Medicine, London 2009.

Box 14.2 Personal audit

You identify that you often require two attempts to intubate trauma patients after rapid sequence induction of anaesthesia. On review of your logbook, you and your trainer notice that your first attempt usually does not involve the use of any adjuncts. You decide, with your trainer, that you will use an intubating bougie for the first attempt in all trauma cases and will continue to monitor your practice.

Departmental audit

Departmental audit is essential for all disciplines involved in emergency airway management. For example, intensivists may wish to examine the process of care for emergency intubations occurring outside the emergency department or the intensive care unit, where equipment provision and expert assistance may be sub-optimal.

Departmental audit facilitates an ongoing process of quality control, and ensures that all emergency airway practitioners are achieving an acceptable standard. It also highlights any equipment or staffing deficiencies, e.g. the availability and use of capnography for all intubations. Data from a departmental audit can also be entered into a national database, which may help in the establishment of national audit standards.

A core data set has still to be agreed; however, an example is given in Box 14.3.

Box 14.3 Possible core data set

Age and sex of the patient	Reasons for intubation
Diagnosis	Urgency
Patient physiology	Airway assessment
Process of intubation	Practitioner and supervisor
Post-intubation difficulties	Destination

To facilitate audit, the core data should be collected for each case; some individuals may elect to collect additional data for their own purposes.

Although a paper-based logbook is the traditional method, it may be easier to collect data on a computer spreadsheet or database, or on a personal digital assistant: this would also make departmental and national figures easier to collate.

Skills maintenance

Skills maintenance in emergency airway management is an important but contentious issue. Any emergency physician, anaesthetist or intensivist in the

UK will find it hard to see enough clinical cases to maintain competence in the assessment and management of the difficult emergency airway.

Alternative methods are needed to maintain skills: these could include high fidelity human anaesthetic simulator training, which is already used in the airway training of anaesthetists, intensivists and emergency physicians in the UK. Simulators enable a rare but lifelike situation to be simulated in complete safety, with no risk to the patient (Box 14.4).

Box 14.4 Human anaesthetic simulators: possible topics

Difficult airway:	trauma, unexpected failure to intubate or ventilate
RSI-related problems:	malignant hyperthermia, anaphylaxis
Rare clinical issues:	profound hypovolaemia, upper airway burns

---

Simulation is highly effective for developing the non-technical aspects of airway care and resuscitation, such as prioritization and team leadership. However, the small number of centres and the increasing demands placed upon them limits the availability of simulator training in the UK.

Alternative methods of skill maintenance include regular sessions in hospital operating theatres. Ideally, these should involve operating lists that have a high turnover of patients (e.g. gynaecology, otorhinolaryngology) and those where tracheal intubation and difficult airways are more likely (maxillofacial surgery, otorhinolaryngology).

The increasing use of the laryngeal mask airway (LMA) and other supra-glottic devices has led some to question the usefulness of elective operating lists for gaining experience in emergency airway management; however, they provide an opportunity to use rescue devices, such as the LMA, in a controlled environment.

Regular training in the operating theatre also fosters co-operation between the specialties involved in emergency airway care. This co-operation should be extended further, with regular joint review meetings between anaesthetists, intensivists and emergency physicians to discuss ongoing departmental audit.

Summary

- Continuous audit is essential for all emergency airway practitioners.
- Individuals should contribute to departmental audit and, where appropriate, national audit to ensure good quality emergency airway care.
- Skills maintenance is vital, and may not be assured from clinical practice alone.

Further reading

1 Nolan, J. & Clancy, M. (2002) Airway management in the emergency department. *Br J Anaesth*, **88**: 9–11.

2 Fletcher, G.C.L., McGeorge, P., Flin, R.H. *et al.* (2002) The role of non-technical skills in anaesthesia: a review of current literature. *Br J Anaesth*; **88**: 418–29.

3 Graham, C.A. (2004) Advanced airway management in the emergency department: what are the training and skills maintenance needs for UK emergency physicians? *Emerg Med J*; **21**: 14–19.

Appendix: Emergency airway algorithms

Acknowledgement
Martin Wiese designed the visual layout of all three algorithms.

Emergency Airway Management, eds. Jonathan Benger, Jerry Nolan and Mike Clancy.
Published by Cambridge University Press. © College of Emergency Medicine, London 2009.

Planning for intubation

Assessing urgency

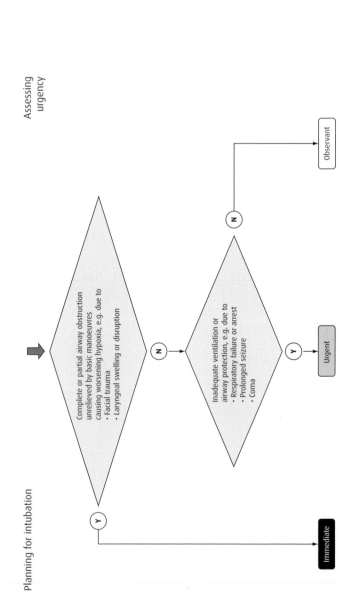

Complete or partial airway obstruction unrelieved by basic manoeuvres causing worsening hypoxia, e.g. due to
· Facial trauma
· Laryngeal swelling or disruption

Y → Immediate

N →

Inadequate ventilation or airway protection, e.g. due to
· Respiratory failure or arrest
· Prolonged seizure
· Coma

Y → Urgent

N → Observant

Predicting
difficulty

History	Ask about previous airway problems
Anatomy	Look for prominent upper incisors, receding chin and macroglossia
Visual clues	Obesity, facial hair, age
Neck mobility & accessibility	Presence of cervical spine immobilization or disease, such as rheumatoid arthritis
Opening of the mouth	Intubation may be difficult if <3 fingers
Trauma	Assess for possibility of anatomical disruption and blood in the airway

Difficult airway predicted?

Y — Call for help

N — Proceed with caution

Preparing

Positioning	
Equipment	Trolley, suction, oxygen delivery, airway adjuncts, laryngoscopes, tracheal tubes, bougies & stylets, drugs, ventilation system and failed intubation equipment
Attach	Oxygen and monitoring: pulse oximetry, capnometry, NIBP and ECG
Check	Resuscitation, brief history, IV access and neurology
Help	Number and abilities of available personnel

Algorithm one Patient assessment and preparation for intubation.

RSI algorithm

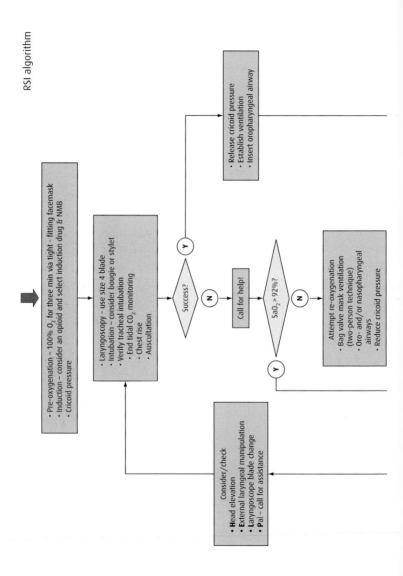

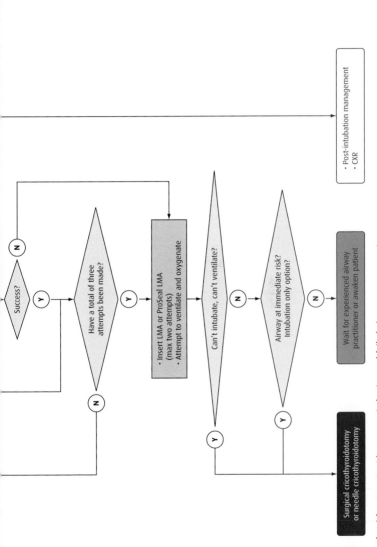

Algorithm two Rapid sequence induction and failed airway management.

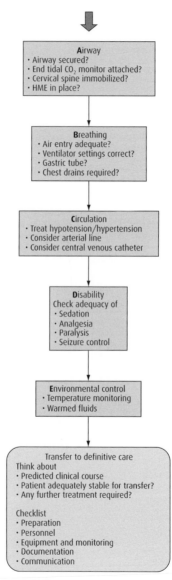

Algorithm three Post-intubation management.

Index